Reiki :
The Science of Healing

Published by :
Lotus Press Publishers & Distributors

Reiki : The Science of Healing

By
Dr. Rajeev Sharma
M.D., D.Lit.

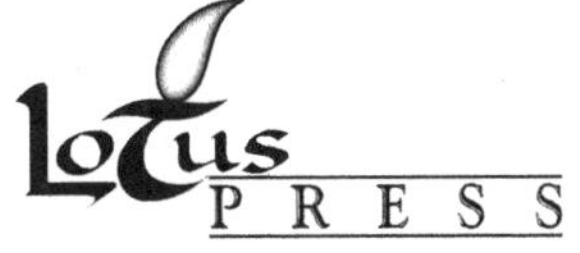

4735/22, Prakash Deep Building
Ansari Road, Darya Ganj,
New Delhi - 110002

Lotus Press : Publishers & Distributors
Unit No. 220, 2nd Floor, 4735/22, Prakash Deep Building,
Ansari Road, Darya Ganj, New Delhi- 110002
Ph.: 98118-38000
• E-mail : lotuspress1984@gmail.com
www.lotuspress.co.in

Reiki : The Science of Healing

ISBN: 81-8382-136-7

Printed & Published by : **Lotus Press Publishers & Distributors,** New Delhi-02

PREFACE

Reiki means treatment by energy of our body through hands. This is an ancient science which has its roots in India, though it got recognition in Japan and China.

Reiki can not be learnt without practising yogic exercises, meditation, pranayama, energizing chakras etc.

In this book, I have tried my best to provide knowledge on all these topics, which will help you in becoming a good reiki practitioner. It is advised that you should have consultation from any renowned reiki practitioner for proper and practical guidance. Our body has a lot of energy and by proper practice we can attain the reiki master level.

If you have any querries you can write to me on: sharmarajeev108@rediffmail.com.

–Dr. Rajeev Sharma

A Brief About
Dr. Rajeev Sharma

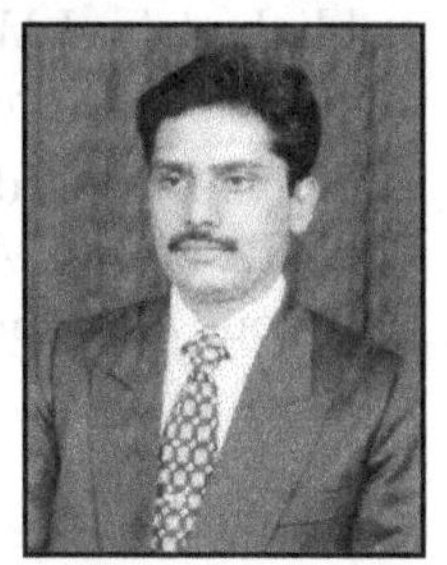

Dr. Rajeev Sharma is an eminent consultant of Homoeopathy,Yoga, Naturopathy and Alternative Medicine in India. He has written more than two hundred books (200) in Hindi and English and around one thousand five hundred articles which have been published in various newspapers and magazines. He is also an Editional Board Member of the prestigious *Asian Homoeopathic Journal* besides many other newspapers and magazines.

Dr. Rajeev Sharma has written books on ayurveda, homoeopathy, yoga, naturopahty, accupressure, magnetotherapy, water-therapy, massage and aromatherapy etc.

Dr. Rajeev Sharma has written books on all major ailments like diabetes, hypertension, obesity, stomach and respiratory disorders, E.N.T. disorders, female and male disorder, UTI disorder sexual disorders, paediatric problems, headache, stress and other mental problems etc.

Dr. Rajeev Sharma is Medical Advisor to Ralson Remedies (a homoeopathic manufacturer), and Dixit Pharmacy (Ayurvedic Manufacturer), Medical Examiner at the Life Insurance Corporation of India. He has received several prizes for his outstanding achievements. He has been awarded the *Best Author prize in Hindi* by the Home Ministry and Ministry of Health and Family Welfare, Government of India and *Sarjana Puraskar* by *U.P. Hindi Sansthan,* Lucknow. He has delivered talks on All India Radio and lectures on Alternative Medicine in various Government and Non-government Organisations. He has written at Advt. Scripts for the products of several companies.

Dr. Rajeev Sharma is also a social activist. He has worked a lot against Addition and Prevention of AIDS. Now-a-days, he is working to check the population growth of India with an NGO called 'Nav Chetna Manch'. He has worked for pollution control and human rights too and has received the World Human Rights Promotion Award. His name has been published in *LIMCA BOOK OF RECORDS* 2005. He has developed one websites too :- www.newkamasutra.com

He is all india president of an NGO "UTKRISHTA-BHARAT" (an All India Association of Socio-Cultural-Religious and Sports Activities).

CONTENTS

1

HUMAN BODY SYSTEM

There are eight basic systems of the human body

(*i*) Skeletal System
(*ii*) Muscular System
(*iii*) Circulatory System
(*iv*) Nervous System
(*v*) Respiratory System
(*vi*) Digestive System
(*vii*) Excretory System

We shall discuss these one by one.

Digestive System

The food that we take comprises proteins, sugars and starches, vitamins, salts, fats and oils. Only a part of these substances is useful to the body and the rest, which is indigestible, must be get rid of. The foot is broken up by the teeth and after getting mixed with saliva, it is swallowed. Saliva is an alkaline fluid which is also common to the air passage at this level. It then passes into the gullet. Like stomach and intestines, the gullet is a muscular organ and can force the food along if necessary. With the help of the muscle, a man can drink even if he is standing on his head. About nine inches long, the gullet ends in the stomach. It is here that the second stage of digestion takes place.

From this position the food reaches stomach which is a hollow muscular organ lined by a glandular mucus membrane which secretes the gastric juice containing hydrochloric acid, salts, pepsin and water. The stomach mixes the food well by moving it round and round. At one stage the proteins are changed to a form in which they can pass through the stomach well and be absorbed, at once, ready to nourish the body.

Starches and proteins are now acted upon, though not digested completely. Fat and oil are broken up and oil is set free. In the stomach, digestion may take two to three hours. The food then goes to small intestine which is a long tube which, when uncoiled, may measure about one feet. Here, we have to consider the action of three different digestive juices, e.g., the pancreatic juice, the bile generated by the liver and the intestinal juice, which is the secretion of the small glands of the bowel lining. Food passes through the intestine and finally nutrients are absorbed and carried into the blood. The bile and the pancreatic juices are produced by the liver and pancreas respectively.

Liver is the largest organ in the body, which is situated just underneath the diaphragm rather on the right side. Its weight is about three to four pounds. There are fine tubes in the liver called bile ducts into which the cells of the liver secrete vile, and the bile ducts join together and form Hepatic duct which carries the bile to the duodenum (also known as first part of small intestine).

Bile is a yellow fluid, containing mucus, water and some salts (called bile salts). It acts on the fats and oils and breaks them up into very small particles.

Liver is also a storehouse for sugar which it puts in the blood, when it is required by the body. About seven inches long, there is another large gland reddish in colour and known as Pancrea's. It lies behind the stomach, and tube from it called the Pancreatic duct enters the intestine near where the bile duct enters. The pancreatic juices act on the protein the starches and the fats.

The intestine is an organ of digestion as well as of absorption. The food, now digested, can pass through the walls of the intestine and is taken into the blood. It is then distributed all-over the body. Food remains in the small intestine for about 12 hours and is slowly passed on towards the large intestine.

The large intestine is a 6 feet long tube. It is little concerned with the digestion or absorption of food, for more of this has already been done. Food remains here from 24 to 36 hours. Due to loss of water, the material in the large intestine now hardens as it reaches the rectum. Finally, the ingestible remnant is turned out.

Excretory System

It comprises the kidney, skin, lungs and bowels. The system is designed to help get rid of the waste matter in the body when all juices have been extracted from the digestive food. There are two kidneys, situated one on each side of the backbone in the small portion of the back or loin. It has the renal artery which brings blood to it and the renal vein which takes it away. In addition, there are the usual nerves, the lymphatic vessels and the ureter, the tube that takes urine from the kidney to the bladder which is the reservoir for urine.

Urine, a pale yellow fluid, carrying the waste nitrogen from our protein foods, and also mineral salts, secreted into the two kidneys. The kidney may be regarded as a pair of filters, through which about 2 pints of blood circulates every minute. In fact, the whole blood in the body passes down to the kidneys in five to six minutes. Urine is propelled down along the ureters from the kidneys to the bladder by successive veins of contraction in the muscular walls of these channels.

The bladder is an elastic membrane serving as temporary reservoir for urine, secreted by the kidneys. The normal adult capacity is about 1 pint. The urine is discharged into the bladder in intermittent jets every 20 seconds or so. The outlet below the bladder is normally closed by a tight ring of muscle called sphincter. In emptying, the bladder contracts and the sphincter relaxes to allow efflux of urine.

Another important agent for excretion of the waste material from the body is skin. It has two layers, the top one called the epidermis and dermis or true skin below the epidemics.

The latter is richly supplied with blood vessels. The skin is designed to:

- protect the body;
- act as an organ of excretion by means of sweat glands. It thus helps to regulate the temperature of the body and;
- to give the sense of touch.

The skin has hair and sense organs. The latter are little lumps in the dermis which are nerve ending. They report to the nervous system when anything comes into their contact. The skin also has two kinds of glands, the Sebaceous glands, which secrete an oily substance serving as lubricant to the skin and the sweat glands which make the skin as an excretory organ. The function of the latter is to take up sweat from the blood and pour it out on the skin. Though mostly water, the sweat contains, salts, fats and tiny bits of skin.

Bowels are the intestines, both large and small, which serve to complete the digestion of food and to allow its absorption into the blood stream. The useless or undigested food remains are gradually moved onwards and are hardened in the large intestine wherefrom they are ready to be thrown out. The failure of the bowel function is called constipation.

Lumps comprise two elastic spongy masses, almost filling the chest cavity. These are import agents to cleanse the system of impurity. Lungs throw off carbon dioxide, water (in the shape of vapour) and also some organic matter.

They are, therefore, organs of excretion in addition to being the organs of respiration.

Respiratory System

This system comprises lungs and the passages leading to them.

The purpose of respiration (breathing) is the entry and exit of air to and from the lungs. The object of breathing is to bring oxygen of the air into contact with the blood with the purpose of (a) giving some oxygen to the blood and (b) taking out waste products from the blood.

The air, in going to the lungs, has to go through various passages. They are nose or mouth, and the larynx or voice box.

We breathe through nose or through mouth. There are two passages leading downwards from nose and mouth into the body one takes food and water to the stomach and the other takes air to the lungs.

Larynx or voice box is commonly known as "Adam's Apple" and can easily be felt in the throat. It is a cavity (inthroat) holding vocal cords. Vibration of cords produces vocal sounds. The air passes from the voice box to the lungs by means of wind pipe which is about four inches long and one inch wide. The wind pipe at the lower end, is divided into two branches that go to the lungs.

The functioning of the lungs has already been described while discussing the Excretory System. The functioning of lungs as the respiratory organ is slightly more complicated. In the lungs, the air gets very close to the blood, that comes from the whole body through heart. The impure blood, dark red in colour, has too much carbon dioxide in it. This blood comes from the tissues, which have taken the oxygen from it but have loaded it with carbon dioxide. In the tissues, oxygen is used every minute to burn up the food material, resulting in production of considerable quantity of carbon dioxide. The lung's function is to reverse this state of affairs, *i.e.*, restoring its oxygen quota and expelling the excess carbon dioxide. Thus the venous blood (the impure blood) is rendered arterial (bright red in colour) in its passage through the lung capillaries. It goes back to the heart and is ready to do its work again. The fresh oxygen, taken by the blood all over the body, is picked up again by its muscles which need it for their normal functioning.

Circulatory System

This system comprises the blood and heart and their functions. The blood is continuously propelled by the contraction of the heart and is derived into the arteries. The arteries are elastic tubes which by their recoil aid the distribution of the blood to all parts.

The blood is a clear fluid comprising innumerable solid bodies called corpuscles. The corpuscles are of two kinds: red and white and are cellular shaped. The red corpuscles carry haemoglobin which constitutes protein and a little iron.

When combined with oxygen haemoglobin forms a bright red substance. The white corpuscles are living organisms, small jelly like creatures each with a nucleus. They are of great importance as they eat up the disease germs that enter the body. They are capable of independent movement in the blood stream and within the tissue and can swallow up dead bacteria and foreign particles.

The main functions of blood are the following:

- It carries oxygen to every part of the body that requires it.
- It carries impurities from all parts of the body to the excretory organs namely the lungs, the kidneys and the skin.
- It carries food from the digestive system to all tissues.
- It carries heat to all parts of the body.

The heart is a hollow, muscular and somewhat conical four chambered force pump enclosed in a fibrous bag. It is situated in the chest between the lungs and weigh from 10 to 12 ounces. The heart is divided into two parts by a wall running from top to bottom with no direct connection between the parts. These parts are themselves divided into parts, upper and lower but have valves between them. The upper portions are called Auricles and the lower ones Ventricles.

When the blood reaches the tissues it loses all its oxygen and is loaded with waste materials especially carbon dioxide from the tissues. The impure blood reaches the heart by means of capillaries and veins. With the beat of the heart, it enters into the Right Auricle and then to the Right Ventricle from where it is taken by the pulmonary Artery to the lungs. In the lungs capillaries, the blood comes into contact with oxygen and is purified (oxygenated). The purified blood is now brought back to heart by means of Pulmonary Vein. It now enters the left Auricle and when auricles are contracted during the heart beat, the blood passes to the left Ventricle and then commences its journey again to all parts of the body. Thus with the contraction of right and left auricles, the venous blood from the body and aerated (oxygenated) blood from the lungs is pumped into their respective ventricles. And when the right and left ventricles contract, venous blood is pumped into the lungs and the aerated blood into the main vessels. These rhythmic contractions and dilations followed by an equivalent pause are called pulse or heart beat.

Muscular System

Muscles are attached to the bones and consist of bundles of fleshly fibres, capable of contraction or shortening. When required such contractions help the various limbs of the body to move. The muscles are of two kinds namely the voluntary muscles whose movements are controlled by human will and the involuntary muscles which perform their function without any conscious effort of the will. These include the heart, the muscles of the stomach and those of the intestines. Their movements are rhythmic and we are not conscious of their action.

Skeletal System

The bony skeleton supporting the human body is constructed to strengthen the muscles which produce movement in the body to give shape. The forelimbs of the human body are supported by bones forming a shoulder girdle and similarly the leg bones are connected to others forming a pelvic girdle. Ribs connected to the backbone (including those connected to the breast bone) serve to protect certain internal organs, including the heart and the lungs. Man's structural superiority over other animals is due to the straight femur or thigh bone and the erect poise of the head.

The above features enable the man to' walk in an erect position so that his hands are tree to perform other functions. These structural advantages and the formation of his skull and lower jaw are responsible for an increase in brain power and intelligence in man, as compared with the other animals.

The human system consists of 206 bones of various sizes. The bones are composed of cells, which are softer in early childhood than in adult life. Where bones meet there is a joint which may simply be an immovable joint as in the bones of the skull or may be movable joint as that of the knee. The movable joints are necessary for the motion of human body.

Nervous System

It is the most important system as it commands rest of the body what to do and how to work together. While the central nervous system resides in the skull and the spine, the nerves are spread all over the body. The nervous system of a man is a network pervading the whole body, having two way connection with the central control and enabling the individual to give a coordinated response to any stimulus from outside. Thus nerves that carry the messages to the muscles with orders to perform a particular action are called Motor Nerves.

The brain is the chief centre of the nervous system and is contained within the skull. The brain substance consists of grey and white matter. The grey matter forming a thin, superficial layer (cortex). It consists of three parts: (a) the cerebrum or bigger brain, which governs our consciousness, thought, emotions, will, sight, hearing, sensation of pain and memory through the grey matter, (b) the cerebellum or the smaller brain is connected with

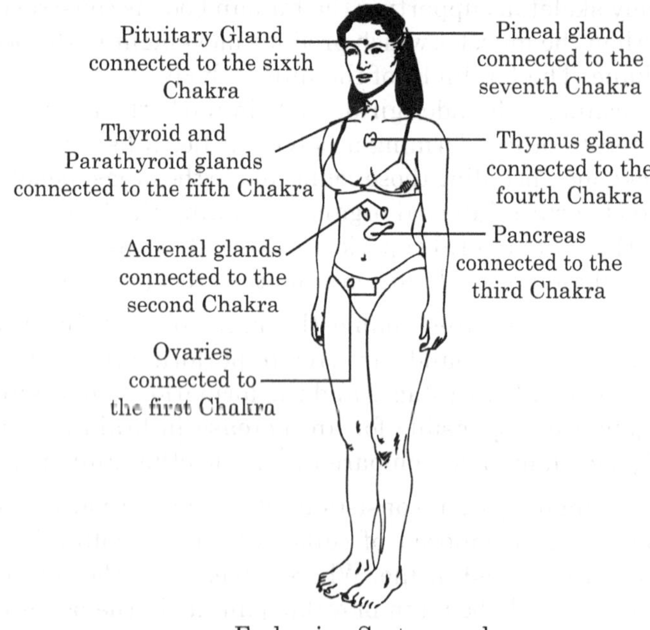

Endocrine System and Position of Chakra

the coordination of the actions, nervous and muscular, by which the movement of the body are carried on, (c) Medulla Oblongata houses the centre of nervous tissue connected with reflex action consisting of movements that take place automatically, such as breathing or walking.

The spinal cord consist mostly of nerves. This is like a continuation of the medulla and runs down the back, surrounded by the bony arch of the spinal column. This organ is capable of making simple decisions, called the reflex action.

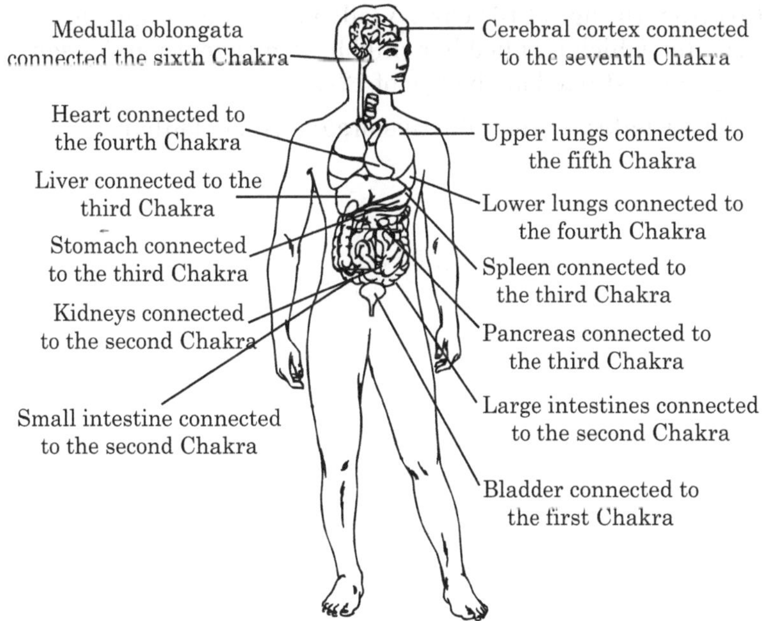

The Human Anatomy and Position of Chakras

Reproductive System

Reproductive system includes external and internal sex organs. A Reiki practitioner should control its over induegence in sex.

The chief female organs are:

Vulva, Hymen, Larger labia, Minor labia, clitoris; There are external genitol organs. The internal organs include: Vagina, Uterus, Fallopian tube, Ovary, Cervix, Bortholin gland.

The chief male organs are:

Penis, Testicles, Scrotum; These are external organs. The internal organs include: Prostate gland, seminol vesicle, vas deferans.

Urethra also play an important role in both male and female, during sex.

Sex is performed for pleasure and progeny. For progeny, it is must but for pleasure this may be controlled.

The Secretion of harmones and development of sex organs start from the age of 13 years. A lady menstruates upto 36 years normally, which is called her child bearing age. In males semen secretion is started at the age of 12-14 years.

The Chakra of reproductive organs is mooladhara.

2
HISTORY OF REIKI

Reiki's origin is tracked back to Tibet thousands of years ago. The ancient cultures in southern India also indicate the origin of Reiki. In ancient times, this science was handed over for initiation after a long preparation. As such, the spread was extremely limited. In the mid 19th century Doctor Mikao Usui who worked in a Christian school was questioned by students as to how healing takes place by simple touching or laying on of hands. Dr. Usui unable to explain or demonstrate, set to find out the truth himself. In the course of investigation he studied the Lotus Sutra (the last sermon of Buddha). He found a formula of mystic symbols in the Lotus Sutra and also found that through the process of initiation, the symbols are empowered to tap the cosmic pool of energy (Reiki) which accelerates the near no process in living organisms. Dr. Usui personally experienced the peak of consciousness, and in depth understanding and the dynamics of its working, when he undertook a fast for 21 days and mediated. Thereafter he travelled extensively to spread the use of Reiki and initiate others into the path of Reiki, the cosmic pool of energy.

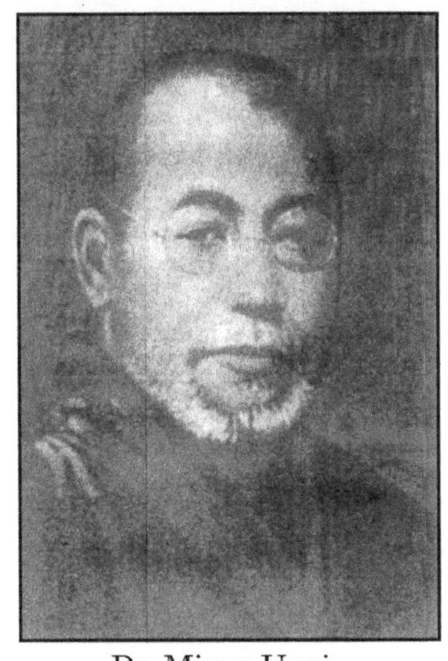

Dr. Micao Usui
(He rediscovered Reiki)

In 1920, Dr. Hayashi joined the tradition and a clinic was set up in Tokoyo. In 1933, a young woman named Hawayo Takata practiced Reiki for nearly 30 years in Honolulu and also initiated people into Reiki in America. However, from just after 1970 till her death in 1980 realising the need to continue the tradition, she finally taught the initiation process, so that the tradition could continue. Some of those initiated by Hawayo Takata have subsequently been responsible for the initiation of other masters who in turn spread Reiki around the world.

3
REIKI: WHAT IT IS?

Reiki is a Japanese word. The word Reiki means universal life energy. It is that power which acts and lives in all created matter. The word has two parts–Rei describes the universal, boundless aspect of this energy and ki is the vital life force energy which flows through all living beings.

We in India know it as Prana and in China it called Chi. In Islamic countries it is known as Barraka. Russian researchers called it Bioplasmic energy.

Since ancient times healing methods based on the transfer of this universal, all pervailing life energy, have existed. This energy which bringsforth all life in the universe and nourished it has been used for healing for centuries. Thousands of years ago the Tibetans already possessed knowledge about the nature of spirit, energy and matter and used this knowledge to heal their bodies and harmonise their souls. This knowledge was there in India and also in Japan and China. We are all familiar with healings done by Gautama Bhuddha, and Jesus Christ and many other spiritual masters who healed others by their touch.

This knowledge was kept secret and was available only to very few people, usually priests who passed it on to their disciples by word of mouth.

All of us may have experienced this energy in some ways. Every time we got hurt and automatically kept our hand on art of the body and felt some relief or when our mother's hand on our forehead when we were ill and we felt better because of her soothing touch.

Dr. Mikao Usui a Japanese missionary, rediscovered this knowledge and the thousand year old tradition of healing in 2,500 year old Sanskrit sutras at the end of the 19th century. He is the one responsible for making it available to all of us again.

Let us find out what is this universal life energy. It is an invisible energy that infuses and permeates all living and non living things. It is pure infinite and limitless. It is odourless and tasteless and we are sustained by it. With every breath we absorb it and yet we are not aware of it.

Modern day scientists are aware of the 'vitality' which pervades all existence. The latest developments in quantum physics and supergravitation theory describe the existence of a standardized, perfectly balanced field of pure intelligence which forms the basis of all creation. This is what wise and enlightened men have said throughout the centuries. They talk about a state of being which contains all creation and from which all life arose. This energy is all around us and it affects our body, mind and our emotions. This energy lives in all things, and this universal energy flows through our hands when we treat some one with Reiki.

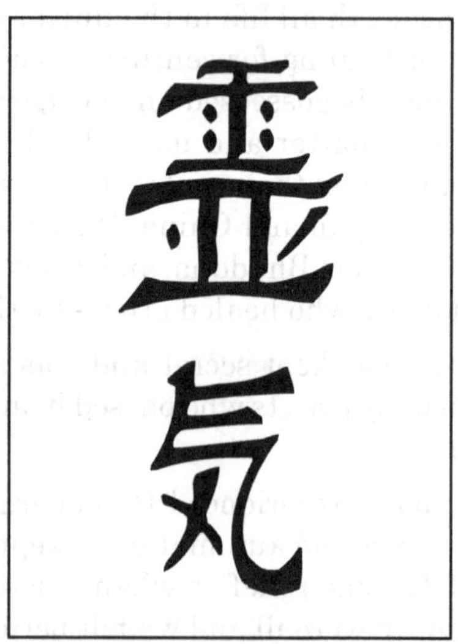

Japanese form of the word Reiki

Researchers in the U.S.A. using various methods including Kirlian photography found that Reiki energy enters the healer through the top of the head (Grown chakra) and goes out from the hands. When the hands are placed on the part requiring healing the energy is drawn to that part and this amplifies the body's self–healing mechanism. This energy increases when treatment is being given.

The Usui system of Reiki is a simple and natural healing method and it is also the most effective way of transferring this universal life energy for healing. Once a person's energy channels are opened up and cleared of obstructions during the Reiki attunement he or she becomes a channer for Reiki, life energy will flow through his/her hands of its own accord and he/she will have this ability for life. Reiki attunement connects the channel to this limitless source of energy. Thus the healer not only receives and increase in this energy for his own healing but is able to canalize this to others by his/her touch and heal them. Reiki healing is all holistic in nature. It brings healing to all levels of our existencey physical, emotional and spiritual.

The healer is only a channel for this energy, it is not his own. This energy passes through him when he lays his hands on a person and leaves him strengthened and harmonized afterwards. Reiki also makes its way to the area of the body which requires treatment. Reiki knows where and how and how much a patient needs it without our being able to add to or subtract from the effect it produces.

Reiki is experienced as love. A loving warmth like one feels with his mother. Love is a uniting power which leads to a state of oneness with the whole of creation.

Reiki can lead us back to this state of health or wholeness (holiness). It is truly a holistic healing method. Reiki healing dissolves our limiting thoughts and moves us towards acceptance of all aspects of ourself. This is a transformational state in which we live in balance and harmony with our environment and our own self. In this transformed state we stop complaining. we experience more vitality, self acceptance, creativity, intuition and clarity.

Reiki has nothing to do with spiritualism or the occult. It has nothing to do with the calling up of ghosts or demons, and it is not hypnosis or any other kind of psychological technique. In Reiki treatment use is made of a neutral, concentrated form of cosmic energy.

A Reiki practitioner requires no special kind of faith or belief. It is used by people of many faiths and religions.

There are two ways in which an individual can benefit from Reiki.

By Going to a Reiki Healer for Healing

A Reiki healer can be anyone who is a Reiki channel and has completed either the first or both first and second degree of Reiki. In a Reiki healing session the patient will be asked to lie down comfortably with eyes closed in a quiet healing room. There may be soft soothing music being played. The healer will then gently place his/her hands on the patient at different places in the front and back. The session may take half an hour to one and a half hours depending upon the number of points to be covere 'd'. During this session the patient will feel a wonderful deep relaxation and patient may even fall asleep. He/she will feel a gentle soothing warm sensation coming from the healer's hands. Sometimes the hands will become very warm. At the end of the session the healer will feel very calm and relaxed and experience a lot of relief. He may take as many sessions as he wants but a full course of healing take 21 days. In some conditions more sessions may be required.

By Learning Reiki

For this an individual will have to go to a Reiki master and attend a Reiki course.

Reiki I is the basic course for beginners. This course is, conducted over one day or two days depending on the group size. There are no special qualifications for attending this course. Anyone above the age of 10 years can attend.

In this course the student receives the Ist degree attunement and is also taught the positions where Reiki is to be given. Some meditations and visualization exercises are also done during the course. From this point the student is able to canalize this energy and is a Reiki practitioner.

Reiki I, sessions are primarily for self healing and Reiki I, healer can also heal someone else if that person is physically present. This healing is done by placing the hands on oneself or another person. Self treatment is very effective for deep relaxation and relief from stress. It creates a balance in our physical, emotional and spiritual self. If also helps to release suppressed emotions and blocks.

In Reilki II, which is an advanced course, another attunement is done and this substantially multiplies the power to channel this energy. This course should be done after a minimum of 21 day's after the first degree course.

This attunement causes emotional and karmic healing in the person receiving it.Reiki II allows the healer to heal those who are not physically present and send this energy over a distance. Reiki symbols are taught which make this possible. This programme also teaches other powerful techniques for using Reiki.

Reiki IIIa is the master healers course in which another attunement is done which further multiplies the power.

Reiki IIIb is the course that qualifies you to be a teacher. Reiki III is recommended only for those who wish to take up healing seriously and want to make Reiki a major part of their lives.

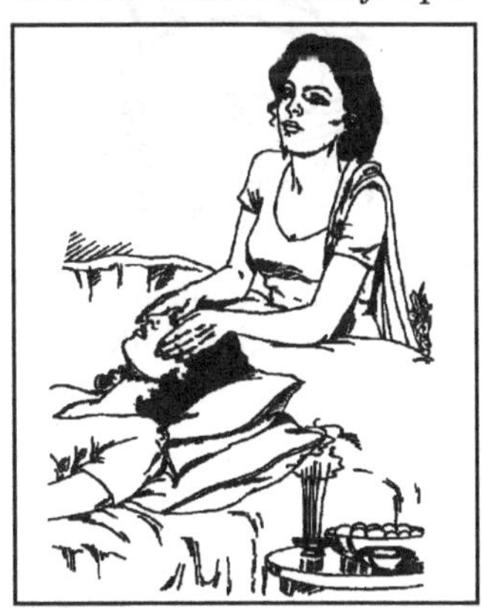

In the first degree of Reiki, a Reiki doctor is giving Reiki to the eyes and cheek of a woman lying on the bed or a table.

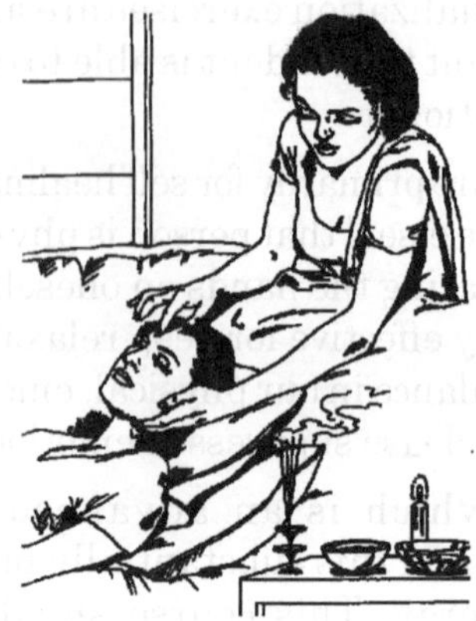

In the second degree, a Reiki doctor gives Reiki by covering/placing her thumb and first finger in the middle of her patient's eyebrows, and with other hand to the patient's left ear and cheek.

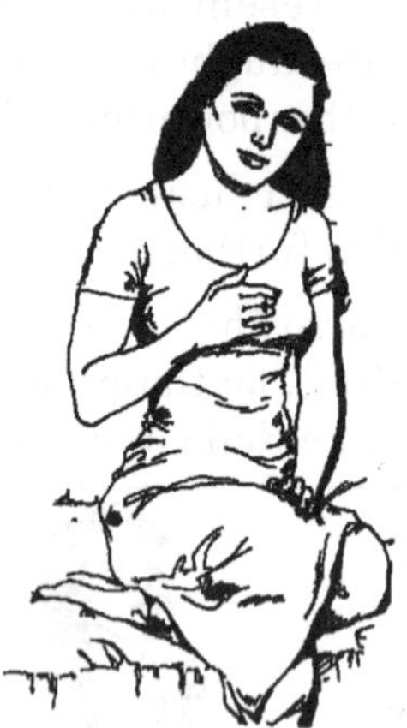

Once the third degree of Reiki is achieved the Reiki healer becomes a master and he or she can give Reiki to herself or himself.

❑

4

SCIENTIFIC POINT OF VIEW

Reiki is energy without any polarities. The energy appears to create harmony and root out disharmony during its physical manifestation i.e. when it assumes the limitations of time and space. In the body, it becomes a form of healing energy.

During the Reiki treatment, a sensation of warmth, the tingling of a needle prick and electrical sensations are felt by the healer. There is another important observation that Reiki turns on automatically without any effort on the part of the healer. The flow of Reiki does not depend on any belief and there is no method of giving Reiki. Once initiated all that you have to do is to place the hands close to the body. There has to be a mere intention of helping by way of treatment. The flow of Reiki is according to the needs of the bodily condition. Therefore, it can either be weak or strong. There is no switching on or switching off of Reiki.

Reiki is not related to any specific religious faith, though the origin appears to be Vajrayana Buddhism (The great Jibetan Master Milerepa was knew to produce psychic heat). The great Yogis in India were also able to even bring the dead to life.

There is no human manipulation of the Reiki energy, which flows according to the body's requirement and works on the levels of both body and mind. Though, the working of Reiki is at best described as mysterious, yet the ancient Masters knew it inner working.

5

REIKI HEALS ON ALL LEVELS

Physical, emotional and spiritual. People (and animals) are not just physical entities. We have a dense or gross physical bodies that we can normally perceive by sight and much. We also have a bioplasmic body or energy body which is invisible and this directs the state of the physical body and our emotional self. Medicine treats only our physical body? Reiki heals us completely, our physical body, our bioplasmic body and our emotional self. Thus Reiki heals the whole person. For example, when a person has a headache and comes to a Reiki healer, the healer will place his hands on the head points and give relief. The headache may have its source in the digestive area and if this is so then the energy goes to this area as well as the head and heals the problem at the source. If the pain is caused by stress then it removes the source of stress. If this person has some other disease or problem that he will not aware of and has therefore not told the healer, Reiki will act here also.

In case of serious diseases the source is usually more than physical and these normally have their roots in emotional trauma. In spiritual despair or negative mental patterns or because of deep resistance to someone or something, Reiki is very helpful in healing all these from the roots.

Reiki raises the level of awareness, makes people more present to life, frees from delusion, stress and disease.

When Reiki energy is channeled it harmonizes the energy body and when the source of the problem is removed, this creates a situation where the body's own capacity to itself is regenerated and then the body heals itself. So clearly, the healer is only a channel and the recipient heals himself with the aid of the Reiki energy that he draws through the healer. Each patient draws in just the right amount of life force energy that he/she needs to release/transform and activate the physical/bioplasmic body so that healing can take place.

Reiki energy heals whatever needs healing, the result can never be predicted. A healer cannot promise a specific result and can only say that the recipient will benefit in some way. Reiki relieves pain, speeds the healing process, stops bleeding, relaxes the receiver and balances the person. The blood pressure drops, respiration slows down and the person becomes peaceful and calm and more energetic. At the end of session a recipient feels as he would feel after a session of deep meditation.

Reiki is helpful in healing almost all conditions. For a person who has no physical or emotional problems, it prevents stress and disease. For those who tire easily as used to happen with my wife, Reiki gives them a capacity to work more without getting tired. Some aches and pains are relieved immediately and chronic problems may take longer to heal. People who get very angry find that their anger has subsided. Sad people become cheerful and in cases of shock and trauma due to grief we find that people come out of it much faster. People with insomnia get almost immediate relief.

Reiki is a very positive energy and can never cause any harm to patient. It can be given to anyone, infant, adult or elderly person. It can even be given to animals. Even when someone is dying it eases the process. In cases of congenital defects or a permanent disability, Reiki may not heal but it will make it easier for the person to live with it. If a body part is lost Reiki cannot replace it but will help the person to adjust to the loss.

Reiki is not being accepted as a part of a trend emerging in western medicine where there is a new paradigm that included mind/body awareness and prevention techniques. Many health care professionals are encouraged to attend Reiki classes to augment their medical skills by leading hospitals in the U.S.A.

Learning Reiki is a major event in a persons life and once a person is attuned his/her life is changed forever. Lots of positive things start to happen after the Reiki attunement. Thus it is an INVALUABLE TOOL FOR A PERSONAL GROWTH.

❑

6
FEELING OF REIKI

In this awareness the shallow 'you' disappear. One has to completely disappear for Reiki to be. The mind ceases, Reiki takes over. Just the attunement does the trick. In otherwords, the presence of Reiki and its descent on you is happening through His grace but only when all the efforts and seekings are dropped, the search has stopped, all the desires have then gone at the receptive stage of the mighty power Reiki. At the time of initiation, it totally inundates you. In that depth, you are not even aware of your existence.

Your own emptiness and the ignition of initiation makes Reiki descend on you. The dancing Reiki symbols enter your crown. Every cell receives it. There is a diving melody.

No words. No sound. It is a totally oneness of the two energies. You are the life force and the great life force Reiki. This is real silence. You remain in the attitude of letting go, utterly relaxed. Reiki has penetrated your being. You find your desires evaporated. The mind is noiseless. Silence dawns. Attachment takes leave of you. You are overwhelmed. You cannot say who You are. That's all.

When Reiki has totally penetrated you, you cannot feel the touch of your body. Your heart is now universal. You have now disappeared and become whole. Just wonder remains. Life is a delight. A gift from Reiki. You don't change but the environment changes favourably for you. Everything becomes extraordinarily beautiful. All the seeds of discard are burnt. You have thrown out all that were inside. This is the result of Reiki penetration and this is the transformation. Let Reiki move to you constantly. Allow it. Surrender to it until Reiki takes possession of you and your heart is no more moved by outer things, only then does the innermost core of your being attract Reiki. The body and mind just become an instrument, a too] for Reiki, the universal life principle. When Reiki moves your heart, everything is fine, everything is beautiful. As I have just started surrender to Reiki. Let it possess you. Let things happen on their own accord. You are living Reiki. You have no private life. You live only because Reiki wants to live through you. It will play its role. You just perform it. No anxiety, no tension, no failure, no frustration, no expectation, no purpose, except to be flooded by Reiki. You are the light of Reiki. Reiki is the beginning, Reiki is the end, Reiki is the goal, the only purpose is to bring the realisation of the void in every heart, give the same to every nook and corner of the world. However, much you hold on, you know you are not a reality. You are filled by the elixir. No more death. You have become Eternal.

The Peak

The supreme possibility is the upward movement of the energy, It is creative. You take a new birth in Reiki. You reach the highest peak of your being. Your consciousness is lifted to the Crown Chakra. This is possible only when the power of Reiki strikes you through initiation by the Master. Then it is a constant upward flow through the great energy? Reiki. This is the real transformation and actual meditation. It is not possible through books, the only answer is? seek a Master.

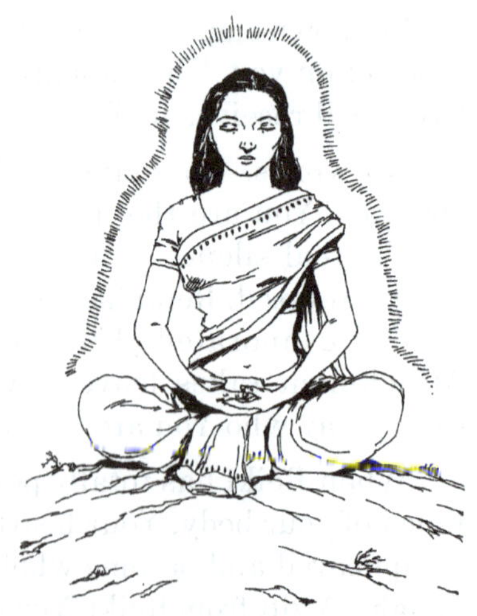

Reiki master, recieving energy present in the universe.

7
HOW DOES REIKI HEAL & WHAT CAN BE TREATED?

How does Reiki Heal

We are alive because life force is flowing through us. Life force flows within the physical body through pathways called chakras, meridians and *nadis*. It also flows around us in a field of energy called the aura. Life force nourishes the organs and cells of the body, supporting them in their vital functions. When this flow of life force is disrupted, it causes diminished function in one or more of the organs and tissues of the physical body.

The life force is responsive to thoughts and feelings. It becomes disrupted when we accept, either consciously or unconsciously, negative thoughts or feelings about ourselves. These negative thoughts and feelings attach themselves to the energy field and cause a disruption,in the flow of life force. This diminishes the vital function of the organs and cells of the physical body.

Reiki heals by flowing through the affected parts of the energy field and charging them with positive energy. It raises the vibratory level of the energy field in and around the physical body where the negative thoughts and feelings,are attached. This causes the negative energy to break apart and fall away. In doing so Reiki clears, straighten and heals the energy path ways, thus allowing the life force to flow in a healthy and natural way.

What can be Treated?

Reiki is both powerful and gentle. In its long history of use it has aided in healing virtually every known illness and injury including serious problems like: multiple sclerosis, heart disease and cancer as well as skin problems, cuts, broken bones, headache, colds, flu, sore throat, sunburn, fatigue, insomnia, impotence, poor memory, lack of confidence, etc. It is always beneficial and works to improve the effectiveness of all other types of therapy. A treatment feels like a wonderful glowing radiance and has many benefits for both client and practitioner, including altered states of consciousness and spiritual experiences.

If a client has a healthy condition, and wants to be treated with Reiki, it is recommended that he should do so under the supervision of an enlightened medical doctor or other health care professional. Reiki will improve the results of all medical treatment, acting to reduce negative side effects, shorten healing time, reduce or eliminate pain, reduce stress, and help create optimism.

❑

8
GIVING A COMPLETE REIKI TREATMENT

Before the client comes you may want to clear and lighter the energy in the room by burning some incense sticks or using an essential oil. Candles are also helpful and create a nice ambiance. Spend a few minutes talking with the client to gain support. Explain the Reiki process, and the hand positions and answer any questions the client may have.

Wash your hands before and after the treatment. Make sure the client and you are comfortable during the treatment. If you sit in an uncomfortable position, it will slow the flow of Reiki. Especially make sure your arms and hands at relaxed. A massage table with chair will make giving a treatment more comfortable.

Before starting the treatment, ask the client to close their eyes, and meditate on being thankful for, and open to, all the healing energies that are coming to his/her. You can also ask them to focus on any pleasant feelings that develop and to let go of distress.

Sit quietly with your hands on your legs doing Reiki on yourself for a few moments. Then draw the power symbol from the top of your head down to spiral in the solar plexus so as to clear, protect, and empower you.

Make the power symbol in the middle of the room, and visualize it on the four walls, ceilings and floor to clear the room of negative energies and fill the room with light. Then say a prayer asking your guides and the client's guides as, well as the angels and all the healing forces of the Universe to work with you to protect the process, and create the most powerful healing possible.

Draw the power symbol on each of your palms and draw all three symbols over the client's heart, or draw the symbols over the client's Crown chakra imagining them going through the crown and into the heart.

Scan. Begin the standard treatment. Remember to draw or visualize the power symbol over any areas that need special attention. Also, visualize the power symbol inside the body within the. organs, or areas that need healing.

Do beaming. This is best done by moving five or six feet away so you are outside the client's aura.

While giving Reiki, meditate on the Reiki energies and on the consciousness of Reiki allowing your consciousness to become one with the Reiki consciousness. Also, your mind will be one with the client's mind when giving a treatment so project positive thoughts to the client during the treatment such as "I know I am healed, I know I am solving my problems" or other affirmations you and the client have formulated.

End the treatment by sealing the client's energy field by drawing the power symbol on the client's solar plexus and covering it with your hand briefly and stating to yourself, " I completely seal this Reiki treatment with divine love and wisdom." Brushing down the aura from the head to the feet also helps to complete the treatment.

After the client has gone, sit quietly doing Reiki on yourself. Visualize the power symbol on the walls and in the centre of the room to clear and protect the room. Your Reiki energies will be high at this time so use them for your special projects, distant healing etc.

Kirlian Photography

Kirlian photography is a technique that allows the etheric energy patterns around living things to be photographed. The process was pioneered by Semyon Kirlian, a Russian Researcher in the

1940's. It is based on a phenomenon known as corona discharge. When an object is in a high frequency electrical field and becomes grounded, a spark discharges between the object and the electrode a piece of film is placed between the object and the electrode and the discharge pattern is captured on the film. When a living thing is used as the object, beautiful colours and patterns seem to follow the pattern of the etheric aura, field of energy surrounding all living things.

❑

9
ADDITIONAL PREPARATIONS

Here are few additional things you can do to empower, the Reiki treatment. Doing them will add an interesting dimension to the treatment as well as make it more fun. You can do them all or just a few. They can also be used in self treatment.

Have the client write out the things that are not working in their life as desired. Include all areas of life (this will cause the problems to come to the surface where Reiki can work more easily

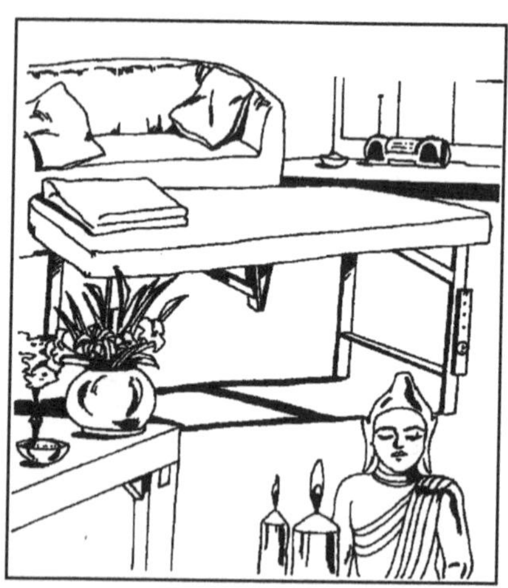

Before you provide Reiki to someone you should clean the room or place which is to be used. Clean cloth on the table, a scented Agarbatti, light music, candle light and a idol of your deity. This all gives a good/favourable atmosphere for this pious job.

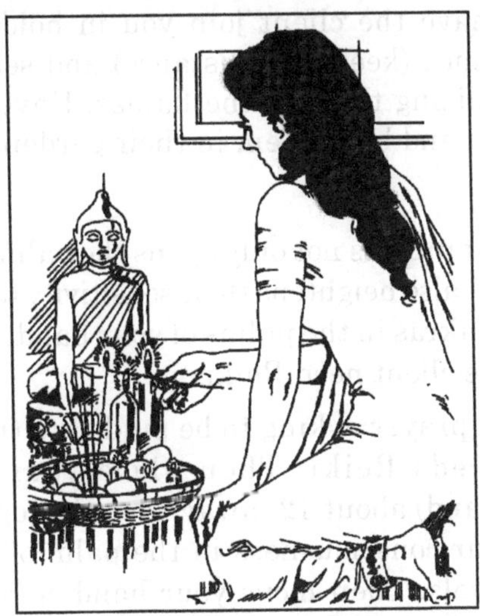

In this figure a woman is lighting candles and agarbattis before the idol of Mahatma Buddha. This way she is preparing the atmosphere to or get achieve Reiki attunement.

on them). On another paper, have them write out the goals and positive results they would like to achieve. Give them a few minutes by themselves to do this.

Then help the client formulate affirmations to heal the problems and achieve the goals. Write them on another piece of paper. Take all three papers and put them into an envelope and have the client hold them while receiving the treatment. Be sure to use the mental/emotional symbol (this symbol opens the subconscious) during the treatment and draw it with your finger on the papers.

During the treatment, have the client repeat the affirmations to themselves. While giving the treatment, imagine you are projecting the affirmations into the client. Remember, during a Reiki treatment the client will be very open to positive suggestions so this is a very powerful process.

Burn the papers in a metal bowl after the treatment. If doing this indoors, find a safe place. Do this as a symbolic ritual. Imagine the flames are transmuting the unwanted conditions into healing and that the goals are being empowered. During the burning, have the client join you in holding your hands toward the flames (keep safe distance) and secretly use Reiki symbols, visualizing them in the flames. Have the client take the ashes home and bury them in their garden.

Scanning

The attunement process not only opens the palm chakras so that Reiki can flow, it also heightens their sensitivity to psychic energy. By using the chakras in the palms of your hands, it is possible to sense where the client need Reiki.

First, say a prayer asking to be guided to the places where the person needs Reiki. Then place your left hand (or nondominate hand) about 12" away from the top of the person's head. Place your consciousness in the palm of your hand and notice how it feels. Then move your hand closer to about you from the top of the head and begin moving your hand over the person's face and moving down toward the feet continuing to remain about 4" away from the body. Move your hand very slowly and be aware of any change in the energy on the palm of your hand. When you feel and change at all, then you will know that this is a place where the person needs Reiki. You may feel coolness, warmth, tingling, pressure, little electric shocks, pulsations, distortion, irregularity or a pulling. The change may be very slight and you may think it is your imagination. However, trust in your experience. Remember when you first begin to practice scanning, your sensitivity may not be developed yet so you need to pay very close attention. As you practice your ability to scan the body will improve. After a while, you may even find you can scan with your eyes and sense where the problems are or you could begin to actually see the distressed areas.

As soon as you find a change in the energy field, move your hand up and down until you find the height where you feel the most distortion. This could be as high as several feet above the body or you may feel compelled to actually touch the body with your hands. Often the best height is found to be about 4" or so.

When you find the right height, bring both hands together at this spot and channel Reiki. Reiki will heal the problem in the aura and also flow into the physical body and work on the organs and tissues connected to the problems in aura.

Remain channelling Reiki at the detected spot until you feel the flow of Reiki subsiding or until you feel the area is. Then re-scan the area to confirm that it is healed if not, you can continue to do Reiki there until it feels complete. Then move your hand down until you find an other area in need of healing and do Reiki there. Continue whoom you have scanned and healted the whole energy field.

Scanning and healing the energy field is very healthy. The cause of most illnesses and other problems is usually in the aura. By treating the aura, you will be working on the cause and also will be healing problem before they get a chance to develop in the physical body. Also once a problem develops in the body, the problem in the aura can become worse. In addition, healing the aura first, helps the person's energy field accept Reiki more completely and allows it to flow more easily to where it is needed when giving a regular Reiki treatment. Therefore, if your are going to do both scanning and a regular treatment, scanning should be done first.

As you interact with the client's energy field, you will become intimately connected to them. You may become aware of the cause of the distortion and the personal problems connected to it. You may also be given insight into? how the problems were created and what the client can do to facilitate the healing. Share this information only you are guided to do so and then, only with loving kindness without judgement. This is sacred work. Always treat the client and the process with great respect.

❑

10
HOW TO TREAT

Treatment should be done in a conducive atmosphere where healer and healee both feel at ease i.e. is quiet, comfortable, serene environment.

Proper hygiene should be maintained i.e. hands properly washed with soap and water before beginning and after finishing the treatment. Reiki is as effective when the hands are kept an inch over the body surface.

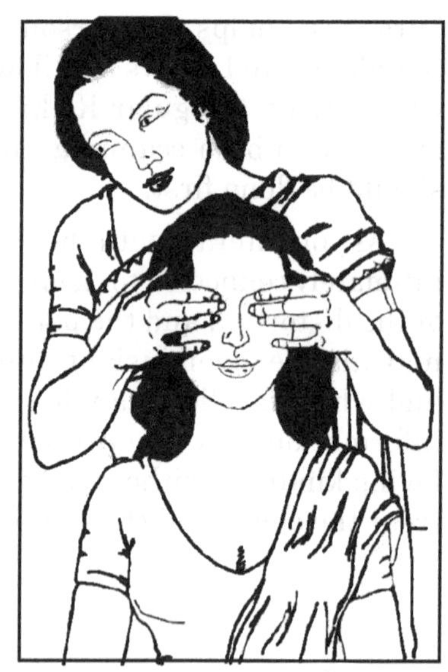

A Reiki doctor, providing Reiki to the eyes to a girl.

The clothing worn by the healer should be loose, without glasses, shoes, tight belts, jewellery etc.

Patient should be made to lie down comfortably his head on pillow, care should be taken that room is cool in summers and warm in winters, patient could use a sheet or blanket to avoid feeling cold, the healer should also be comfortable. Patient's feet should not be crossed.

A brief history of the patients illness, its duration and previous treatments should be taken any past surgery, removal of any organ should also be inquired.

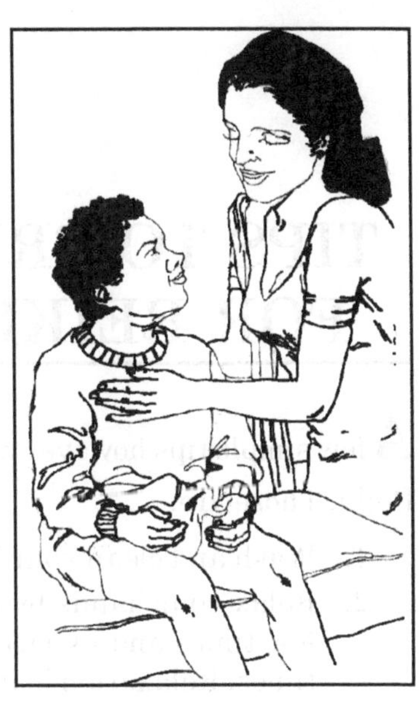

Reiki doctor giving Reiki to a boy by placing her hand on his chest.

Inform briefly about the Reiki and reassure the patient regarding the temporary worsening of the pain of any chronic ailment. This happens as the old malady is brought back to the acute state before being released to where it comes from. If this happens consecutive daily 3-4 treatments, the position of the hands of the healer is important for bringing maximum transfer of energy. Fingers of the hands should be kept together and never slightly curved inwardly.

Begin treating the patient. Spend 8-10 minutes on each Reiki position. With experience the healer can sense rise and fall of Reiki energy and the areas of the body where more energy is required. Begin by treating hand, front and back, treat the organs at their positions even if those were removed by surgery (Presuming them to be present).

❑

11
TIPS TO PREPARE HANDS FOR REIKI TREATMENT

A few simple tips however will prepare your hands better giving Reiki. Those are:

1. Wash and clean your hands properly before giving Reiki.
2. Relax your hands by opening and clenching your fists a few times and by jerking and shaking your hands a few times. Relaxation leads to freer energy flow in hands and more sensitiveness to subtle pranic energy.
3. Bring your awareness to the palm of your hand. This coupled with instructions given in S. No. 1 and 2 activates the hand chakra located at the centre of palms. By activating the hand chakras, one develops the ability to feel subtle energies. This is also called sensitizing the hands. Once your hands are prepared, you can clearly sense the warmth of life energy flowing through them by bringing facing each other as shown in the following fiqure.

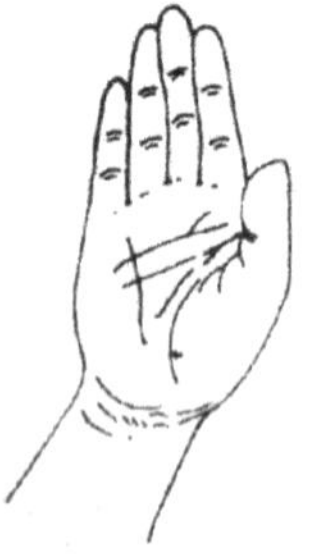

Keeping Thumb and Fingers together

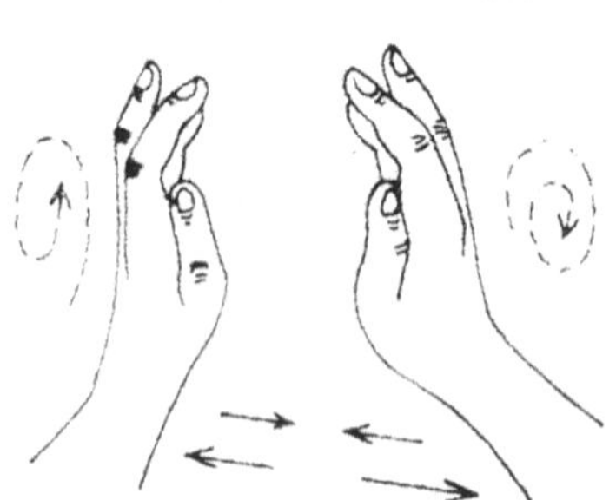

Feeling Pranic Energy

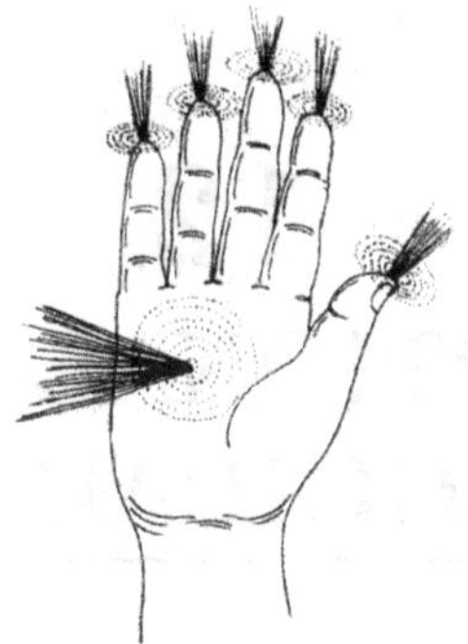

Hand and Fingers Chakras (energy centres)

When giving treatment, it is important to keep your fingers and thumb together. This will concentrate the energy and create a stronger flow. Remember while treating disease try to treat the cause also *i.e.*, treating eyes for diabetic blinders would not suffice. The healee needs to treat on pancreas also for sufficient secretion of insulin. Reiki is drawn by the organs/tissues accordingly to their needs.

Team Treatments

Two healers can plan up to treat the patient as it is quicker simultaneous treatment to back and front on the corresponding areas could be given.

Reiki Finish

At the close of treatment thank the Reiki universal life force, thank yourself for acting as the channel and then the patient for receiving Reiki energy from you. Hold your hands for 30 seconds forstopping the flow of Reiki energy.

❑

12
EMOTIONAL AND PSYCHOLOGICAL HEALING

Many a times, physical illness is a manifestation of deeply buried emotional psychological trauma unresolved childhood issues, which are forgotten. The patient is unaware of cause, but the reaction to life circumstances is as (Negative response) and the person can neither do not, comprehend or come out of negative vicious circle of illness.

Once emotional and psychological blockages are released the physical healing automatically takes place. Remember Reiki is a method hereby the emotions and the body are balanced without the conscious awareness of the patient. Many a time patients weep out, releasing their floodgate of dams of emotion build up in the past which probably were the cause of their illness.

Distance Healing

Distance healing is basically a visualisation exercise. I can be a photograph or a recollection of any sensual impression about the person. Thereafter, it is just sending energy, love, light, strong intention, good imagination of even placing the photograph at the home after where the pictures of Gods and Goddesses are kept in most homes in India. All these are distance healing.

There are many methods. The simplest process is imagining or concentrating on the person, sending the Reiki symbols and seeing the person well returning normal health. Though, hands on healing can be combined, *i.e.*, person receiving absent healing need not know the someone is healing him.

Where the healers' imagination is concerned, Reiki symbols and instructions regarding clearing, visualising Sei-He-Ki at spinal centres are all part of distance healing. There is no need to go into a trance. Simple quietness is enough. Whatever method you use is positive. Concentrate on the person, not on the disease or symptoms. You can repeat distance healing often during the day for the same person, till a specific goal is achieved.

❑

13
BEAMING OF REIKI THROUGH AURA FROM DISTANCE

There are four specific Reiki methods of distance healing:

- Imagine that you are there with the person receiving healing and you are doing, with your imagination, a hands on healing session.
- Imagine the person to have shrunk to a small size hold that image between your cupped palms. You can even see photographs. Send the symbols and hands on healing.
- Imagine your knee and upper hips to be of the person receiving Reiki, The knee being the head, the thigh becomes the torso and your hip represents receiver's leg. Do hands on healing holding the person's image in the mind. The left knee shall represent the person's front and the right his back. This is a wonderful method.
- You can create a surrogate or use the photograph image and do hands on healing on it as though you are doing it for the person. This also work wonderfully.

14
SELF-SCANNING

The scanning process can also be done on yourself. Follow the same steps as above, looking for distortions and administering Reiki when you find them. Self scanning can bring into consciousness aspects of yourself that you were not aware of. You will get to know yourself better and be shown new levels of yourself that need healing.

When you find a distortion in your energy field, ask what happened to create the distortion, and what you can do to help the healing. Remember, be kind to yourself. Accept whatever is shown to you without judgement or blame. Allow yourself to feel your feelings. Be ready to forgive and to let love in. This can be an intimate process, making you aware of deeper needs, increasing your sensitivity and facilitating personal growth.

It is possible to use the distant healing symbol, to beam Reiki to your client from across the room. This can dramatically increase the amount of Reiki flowing through you to the client. It also creates a unique healing process of treating the whole aura at once, before entering the physical body where it is needed.

It is also possible to Beam Reiki directly to a specific area. Just imagine that your hands are like radar dishes and you are focusing Reiki on the area you want to treat. You can also direct it with your eyes by focusing your visual attention on the area.

This process works better if you allow your consciousness to merge with the Reiki consciousness. Simply allow your attention to dwell on your awareness of the Reiki as it flows through you. Focus your mind only on the Reiki. If other thoughts come into your mind, gently brush them away and bring your attention back to the Reiki. By doing this you will enter an altered state that allows the energy path ways.

Reiki flows through to open more than normal. It is also allows your Reiki guides to more easily add their Reiki to Beaming can be done at the end of a standard treatment or it can be done by itself.

A complete treatment can be given to yourself or others with the hands 1" to 4" from the body using the standard and position. Because the hands are in the aura, the Reiki treats the aura before entering the physical body. Illness exists first in the aura before manifesting in the physical body. Treating through the aura will help prevent physical illness before it develops.

The Reiki energies will act in a different, often more powerful way, when using this techniques. They will easily travel through the aura to other part of the energy field? often flowing through and surrounding several areas at one, filling them with warm, loving nurturing energy before entering the physical body at the place. It is needed.

Many people find this method to be more effective while others prefer physical contact. You can use one or the other or you can mix the two. Simply allow your intuition to guide you in deciding where to use physical contact and where to treat through the aura.

In some areas, one must be a licensed medical doctor or have a massage license in order to touch the physical body. If that is the case and you don't have a license, then it is recommended that you do the complete treatment without touching.

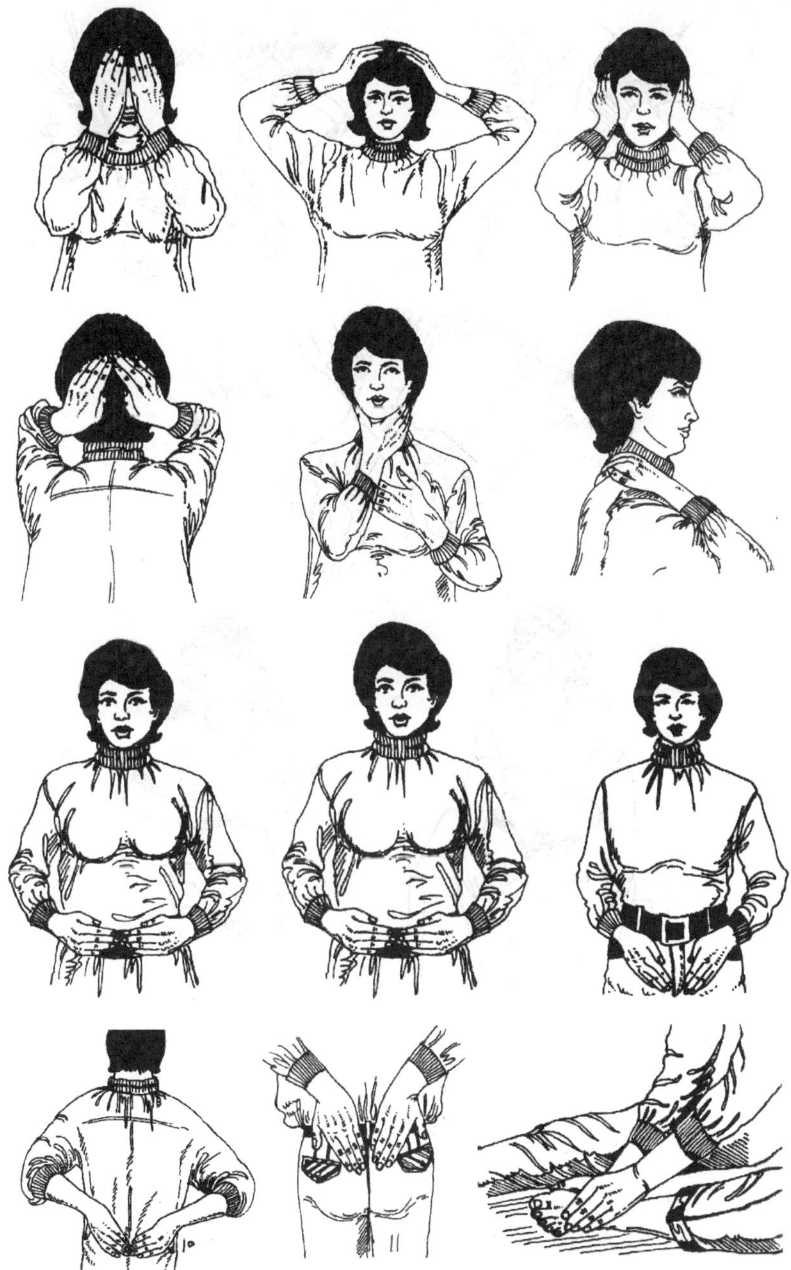

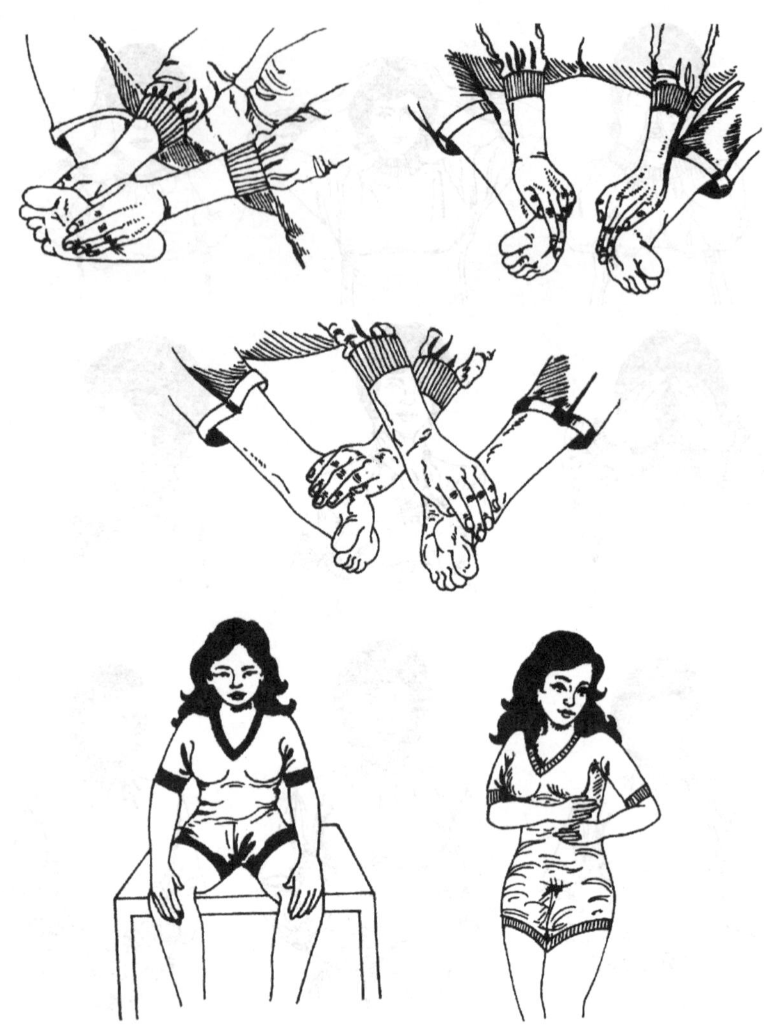

❑

15
REIKI ATTUNEMENT

The Reiki attunement is safe and painless process. It opens and closes obstruction in the body's energy channels. Assume a sitting position with legs stretched forward. Bend the knees and bring the feet together at the perineum. Raise the body onto the heels so that the heels press the perineum. The heels can either point forward or backward. Repeat when all tension has left the legs and feet.

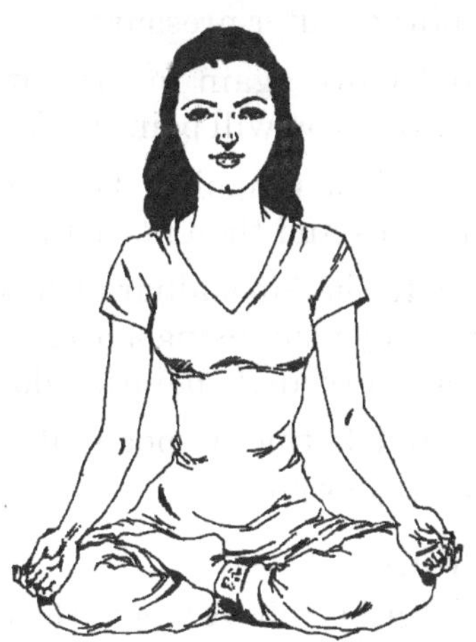

A girl in loose clothing doing pranayama. She is preparing herself for Reiki attunement.

Attunement for Woman

Adopt the above posture. Relax your body completely and close your eyes. Move your awareness to the lower part of the body and focus your attention on the contact point between your heel (or floor cushion) and the opening of the vagina.

- Become intensely aware of the slight but distinct pressure at this point.
- Now become aware of your natural breath.
- Feel or imagine that you are breathing in and out of the pressure point.
- Continue this for ten deep breaths.
- Now bring your awareness inside the body.
- From the point of external pressure, move your awareness in towards the base of the spine.

Follow the natural formation of the vagina, moving up at a slight angle and back towards the spine until you come to the opening of the womb. You are at the opening of the womb, about two/three centimetres inside the body, about two/three cm. above the floor, just below the base of the spine.

Focus your awareness at this point and begin to breathe in the cervix to the point of outer pressure.

Breathe out and move again to the outer pressure point. Somewhere in this area, you will point for Mooladhara Chakra.

If at first you cannot pinpoint the chakra, continue the practice for five minutes and then move to another Asana.

After you do locate the Mooladhara Chakra, mark the spot in your consciousness by visualising a bright yellow square and inside the square, a red triangle pointing downwards.

See this clearly and distinctly spot while you breathe in and out of this internal trigger point.

Attunement to Man

Sit in the posture described above where the heel is pressed into the perineum. Close your eyes and become aware of your whole physical body. Relax completely. Move your awareness to the point of contact between the heel and perineum. Midway between the testes and the anus.

Become intensely aware of the distinct pressure exerted on the perineal body. Centre yourself at the pressure point. Now become aware of your breath. Feel or imagine that you are breathing in and out of this pressure point.

Feel the breath moving through the perineal body, becoming finer and finer, so that it pierces the point where the Mooladhara Chakra is.

You will feel it as a psycho-physical contraction. If you locate the Mooladhara Chakra, mark the spot in your consciousness by visualising a bright yellow square, and inside the square, a red triangle pointing downward.

Visualise this while at the same time breathing in and out of the trigger point in the perineal body. Continue for five minutes. Remember where the pressure point is.

In the case of both men and women, the main clue is to locate the Root Chakra. Once the location is known, contraction of muscles of that area should be achieved and maintained during the whole duration of attunement except then blowing. Breath should be held after inhalation after blowing out on the chakras either in front or at the crow during the attunement.

❑

16
REIKI PRACTICE

Technique–A

- Be aware of your natural breathing.
- Visualise the RAKU symbols? both the thunderbolt form 2nd the wavy form.
- Synchronise the inhalation with mental visualisation of the process of going up the spine, superimposing the symbol RAKU (wavy type). Mentally travel as you breath in from the local portion of the level upto the top portion. RAKU extends from the Medulla travelling down the spine upto the Root Chakra.
- While exhaling synchronise RAKU (thunderbolt pattern) along the spine going down from the Medulla to the Root Chakra.
- Here also synchronising the RAKU symbols, and the spinal column along with the breath should be meticulously followed.

Technique–B

- Sit comfortably in a chair.
- The tongue should be rolled back, mouth closed.
- The breathing is through the nostrils in the expanded throat cavity. It is called belly breathing. The abdomen is withdrawn smoothly and deeply during exhalation and expanded gradually during inhalation.

The eyes are closed and the eyeballs turned upward to gaze, at the point between the eyebrows.

The mind should be kept, simultaneously, (a) at the point between the eyebrows, (b) travelling up the spine or down the spine to synchronise with inhalation or exhalation respectively, (c) To cross all six energy centres from the Root Chakra to the Medulla, (d) To visualize at each centre REIKI symbols and corresponding words. Inhale for a duration of 22 seconds. Without holding the breath exhale for the duration of 22 seconds. Approximately in one hour you breath only 80 times, compared to the normal 800 times. The rate of breath is reduced to one tenth of the normal level.

Inhalation should be synchronised with mentally going up the spine as you cross each centre, stop a while but continue to inhale. Draw the power symbol. Say it three times in your mind. Then go to the next centre. By the end of the inhalation you will be covering the Root Chakra to Medulla in 22 seconds.

- Repeat the same process, down the spine with exhalation for 22 seconds.
- Repeat the same breathing patterns with the emotional healing symbol, the transmission symbol (distance healing symbol), and the Master symbol.

Note: In the beginning the rate of breathing from 800 per hour can be reduced to 200 per hour gradually in the course of 3 to 6 months you can achieve 80 breaths in an hour. Visualisation and the spinal centres alongwith the corresponding words during this process of breathing amounts to the erasing of the Karma with reference to that specific centre.

Technique–C

The breath in and breath out duration should be as discussed above but while inhaling trace the RAKU symbol from the lower portion going upwards and synchronising the same HE the spinal column.

Breath out as discussed before visualising the RAKU symbols downward (thunderbolt forrn) as you exhale RAKU visualisation coincides with the spinal column.

At the end of inhalation, hold the breath and rotate the neck once as described below and then exhale as describe above.

Neck Rotation

At the end of inhalation hold the breath slightly, make a drooping movement so as to make the head drop towards left nipple. Rotate the neck in the anti clockwise direction (one full rotation) and raise the head and drop it towards left nipple as though giving a jerk.

After the neck rotation exhale as described above. The above pattern of breathing i.e. inhalation neck rotation with breath held condition and exhalation is regarded as Pranayama.

- This breathing should be done 80 times an hour. One neck rotation will hardly take less than 3 seconds including the jerky movements towards the left nipple. The Hindu yogis call it Hridyagranthibedha cutting as under the knot of the heart.

❑

17

ROOT CAUSE OF ALL PROBLEMS-ENERGY IMBALANCE

Disease of any kind whether physical, mental or psychosomatic indicates some imbalance inside us. This imbalance is nothing but imbalance in the energy body. It is interesting to note that this life energy or prana is linked both to body and mind. It is an intermediary or bridge between the two and this only explains how physical body affects the non physical mind and how non physical mind affects the body.

Anything happening in the body also affects the mind through the agency of prana. Similarly, anything happening in the mind also affects the body through the agency of prana. Hence body and mind are functioning in a healthy manner, energy or prana is flowing freely and uniformly everywhere. There is no blockage, congestion or depletion of prana anywhere. Hence there is no disease.

However, when body and mind are being misused, functioning unhealthy, abnormally or are overexerted, energy flow becomes imbalanced, *i.e.*, energy becomes blocked and congested at one place, depleted at another place leading to some kind of disease (disease) in body.

Physical Factors Causing Imbalance

Now at the bodily level there are many factors by which we disturb the natural and healthy functioning of energy body. Some of them are listed below:

1. Irregular lifestyle (*e.g.*, sleeping, walking, eating at irregular and odd timings).

2. Overeating, oversleeping.
3. Use of alcohol, smoking (tobacco), tea, coffee, narcotic drugs.
4. Faulty diet (Rajasik & Tamsik foods).
5. Overexertion.
6. Overindulgence in sensual pleasures.
7. Excessive talking/gossiping/roaming unnecessarily here and there.
8. Faulty postures, faulty breathing.
9. Living in polluted, noisy environment. Living in extremely hot/cold/humid environment.
10. Excessive company and mingling with people.
11. Drugs and medication.

In short, if any Rajasik or Tamsik activity disturbs the energy flow of the body then it generates negative energy. On the otherhand, Satwik lifestyle and activities promote the balanced and free flow of prana and generate positive energy. Whatever organs or systems get damaged due to the negative physical factors mentioned above, pranic flow in the corresponding nadis and chakras get disturbed.

Mental Factors Causing Imbalance

As mentioned earlier, just like physical factors, mental factors can also affect energy flow and damage chakras. If we want to sum up all the negative mental factors in two words, which disturb the flow of prana and health of chakras, those two words will be 'Negative thinking'. Now the next question comes' why negative thinking arises'? The simple answer is–not accepting and understanding the things as they really are. The more the gap between the reality of things and your imagination/ assumption about them, the more tense, nervous and anxious you will be.

Because of this huge gap between how things really are and what we imagine them to be, we are continually suppressing, rejecting and fighting with ourselves and outside world. This doesn't allow us to be integrated, whole and complete in our personality. We become a fragmented personality where one portion is going this way, another portion is going that way and third portion is another way. The result is tension and conflict which does't allow energy to flow freely. As per yoga psychology, in such a state our unconsciousness is relatively vast and consciousness not well developed.

So, the first thing to do is to stop suppressing things and start seeing and understanding things from a broader perspective. We should start accepting and integrating everything into our consciousness avoiding nothing. This integration finally leads us to a state of unity, wholeness and completeness. Suppression brings about separation which creates loneliness, discomfort and a feeling of disease. Whatever is suppressed and not integrated into our personality becomes alien to us and a constant source of disturbance. But as we develop, a process of integration takes place among all alienated or conflicting aspects of ourselves leading to increased happiness and satisfaction.

When our consciousness is fully developed, we finally reach that state of enlightenment and equilibrium from which all can be understood, appreciated and accepted. It is also to be noted that when consciousness is not fully developed and integrated, there is lot of egocentric move and selfishness in one's personality and lack of concern for others. But as consciousness gradually becomes expanded and integrated, we become less self-centred with more concern for others. This, in spiritual parlance, is also stated as moving from a state of separation (selfishness) to the state of unity (selflessness).

Now when the personality is not integrated, it is reflected in our behaviour in various forms as mentioned below:

(*a*) Negative emotions (e.g. anger, irritation, impatience, intolerance, fear, anxiety, worry, nervousness, hatred, jealousy, revengeful nature, hurry, overambition, restlessness, depression, sadness, hopelessness and helplessness, lack of confidence, etc.

(*b*) Desires and expectations.

(c) Craving and passion for name, fame, power, status, control, domination.

(*d*) Various 'Vikaras' like greed, attachment, selfishness, ego, etc.

(*e*) Unsteadiness and distractions in mind, inability to focus.

Now the most important question is how these negative mental factors affect our energy body and then the physical body.

The explanation of this question is that these negative mental factors create corresponding vibrations in our astral body. Since astral body is connected to etheric body (or pranic body) at the point of chakras or energy centres, hence corresponding chakras get affected and start malfunctioning. Now the organs to which these chakras feed energy, also start malfunctioning as a result.

The following table shows the relationship between the energy centres (or body part having this energy centre) and corresponding mental factors which influence them.

Mental Feeling

Energy centre which is affected	Energy
1. Inability to love all universally	Heart chakra will be blocked
2. Lack of self-expression, inability to communicate and speak effectively	Throat chakra will be blocked
3. Excessive sex and sensory pleasures	Hara chakra will be blocked
4. Craving for name, fame, ego, power; domination and control over others; aggressiveness, anger, jealousy, hatred impatience, violence, cruelty, harshness exploitation	Solar Plexus chakra will be blocked
5. Compassion, love kindness, sympathy	Heart chakra will be opened
6. Fear, insecurity, feeling threat to digestive disorders, for all unity with creation knees, calves and feet will be affected (Refer Reiki positions)	Root chakra will be blocked
7. Deep–rooted feeling of hurt and guilt	Hara and throat chakras will be affected

8.	Foul speech, shouting, showing disrespect to others	Throat chakra will be blocked
9.	Humbleness and sweetness in talking with love and respect	Throat chakra will be opened
10.	Unsteadiness of mind and eyes	Ajna chakra will be blocked
11.	Inability to forgive enemies	Ajna chakra will be blocked
12.	Extreme helplessness and hopelessness	Paralysis, numbness of arms, hands and leg, Asthma
13.	Over sensitiveness, suppression restricted communication between you and world	Allergy, skin problems (Eczema, Acne etc.)
14.	Steadiness/concentration of mind and eyes	Ajna chakra will be opened
15.	Forgiveness	Ajna chakra will be opened
16.	Greediness, attachment	Hara chakra will be afffected leading to constipation
17.	Disharmony and non adjustment in relationships with partner and other close relatives resulting in disappointment, frustration	Kidneys will be affected
18.	Pent-up aggression, bitterness, hard feelings	Gallstones, kidney stone will be formed.
19.	Overthinking and overplanning	Swadhisthan (or Hara) chakra will be damaged
20.	Fearlessness	Mooladhara chakra will be opened.

Energy Imbalance from Yogic Perspective

In yoga, the energy balance is explained in terms of activity of Ida, Pingala and Sushumna nadis, and it is very interesting to know about it.

Imbalance towards Left Side

As has been explained earlier, Ida nadi (or moon's channel) travels along the left side of the spine starting from the Muladhara chakra and ascending upto Ajna chakra. The qualities assigned to this nadi are Tamoguna, past events and subconscious. It always brings to consciousness the memories of the past. The persons who are left sided (i.e. in whom Ida nadi mostly remains active) are those people who keep on thinking of the past, are very emotional, prefer darkness, avoid meeting people and are introverts. Such persons get various types of diseases of the left side. They become very lethargic, retreating into passivity and self obsession which finally culminates in lunacy, epilepsy, senile decay.

Persons who are left sided should balance it with the right side by activity, work and action, discarding all ideas of self destruction and selfpity. Our left side is represented on the whole left hand.

Imbalance towards Right Side

As has been mentioned, Pingala nadi or the sun channel runs along the right side of spine starting from Muladhara up to Ajna chakra. This nadi has qualities of Rajo Guna. It represents our desire for action (Kriya Shakti). It makes us think, work, plan and organise for the future events.

The symptoms of right sided persons are that they are very aggressive, over ambitious and dominating type. Right sided persons become very dry and lose all soft feelings. They are concerned only for their selfish material achievement and power over others. Blinded by ego, they take pride in exploiting and fooling the world. Such people get diseases of right side, Problems on Pingala nadi result largely from our presumption that it is we who are doing something while in fact all work is done only by Almighty God.

Any extreme physical or mental activity can paralyse our left emotional side and move us on to the right side so that we move into supraconscious (future) where we see visions like those induced by hallucinogenic drugs.

Overactive right side is brought into balance by moving the energy towards the centre, to Satoguna, Our right side is represented on our whole right hand.

Balance at the Centre

When the powers of both left (Ida nadi) and right side (Rajoguna) are brought to balance, we get established in the centre or Satoguna.

The central channel or Sushumna nadi begins at Mooladhara and goes straight up to the highest chakra namely 'Sahasrara'. The qualities of this nadi are Satoguna, present centredness and superconsciousness. It is represented in both the hands. It is thought this channel that we become superconscious and integratd into one whole. When Sushumna nadi gets opened, Kundalini can ascend in this central channel and go right up to Sahasrara chakra leading to our enlightenment. Doing regular meditation in thoughtless awareness (pure perception) and leading virtuous life is vital to opening of Sushumna.

Sushumna nadi is also called the channel of the Eternal present, where the only time is not. In this way, we transcend time and space by opening of Sushumna and Kundalini awakening.

Achieving the Balance of Nadis

In 'Sahaj Yoga' some simple techniques are suggested to achieve the balancing of right and left sides of the body as mentioned below:

(*i*) If a person is right sided then the energy of Ida nadi is raised by making ascending movements of the right hand along the right side and brought to the left side or the person's spine.

(*ii*) If a person is left sided, i.e. apathetic and depressed, then the energy of Pingala nadi is raised by making ascending movements of the right hand along left side of the body and brought to the right side of the person's spine.

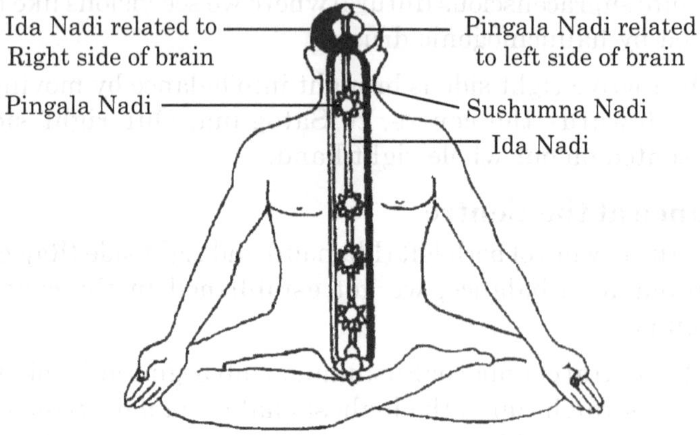

Three Major Nadis

Clearing the Chakras

A chakra could also be cleared by simulating its clockwise rotation with the fingers of the right hand by a healer and asking the patient to keep his right hand on the afflicted chakra and keeping his left hand on the left knee with palms up and fingers open. In the science of prana, left hand is always used for receiving energy and right hand for imparting energy. Now depeding on which side of chakra is afflicted–whether left side, right side, front or back, there can be slight variations accordingly in the healing.

There are other methods of clearing the chakras also, e.g. candling. It clears the chakras on the left side. Here a burning candle is moved up and down on the left side of spine. Similarly, there are other methods for clearing chakras like foot soaking in lukewarm salt water. Right side chakras are normally cleared by cold water treatment in the form of foot soaking in cold water. Foot soaking in river or sea water is said to clear Solar and Hara chakras. Sitting on mother earth or walking barefoot on the earth or grass clears Muladhara chakra. Putting hands on earth or in flowing river water or in lukewarm salt water is equally beneficial for clearing chakras. Salt has the special quality of breaking down the negative energy. Doing concentration or "Trataka" with open eyes on some object especially candle flame helps in awakening the Ajna chakra. Even when in a normal way our mind is focussed and centred in some activity, it helps in activating Ajna chakra. Meditation is the strongest method for energizing Ajna chakra.

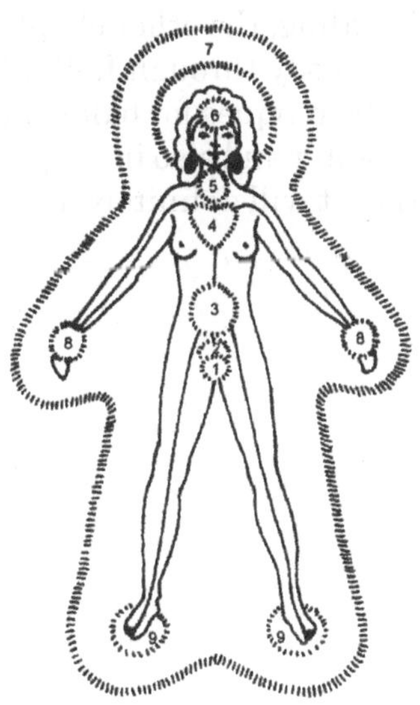

1. Mooladahara, 2. Swadhisthana, 3. Manipura, 4. Anahata, 5. Vishuddha, 6. Ajna, 7. Sahasrara, 8. Lao Kun, 9. Yung Chuan
The Chakra

Yoga science also speaks of reciting (mentally) specific mantras for awakening each chakra. This science is based on matching the subtle frequency of each chakra with subtle frequency of specific mantra so as to create resonance. However, since the subject is Reiki, we won't go into these details in this book.

Another technique of clearing chakra is by strengthening their qualities as mentioned in the table of chakras. As has been mentioned earlier, the chakras which are catching and blocked are only responsible for psychic and physical problems.

One of the easiest method to awaken chakras is to mentally focus your attention (with eyes closed) on them. To increase your concentration on a particular chakra you can imagine that you are breathing through that chakra (*i.e.*, inhaling and exhaling through that point).

All the above information for clearing nadis and chakras is given here only for general enlightenment of the reader. However, since the purpose of this book is to cleanse the energy body through Reiki healing, the other chapters have the details of healing your energy body through Reiki. Nevertheless if you continue to use other techniques for balancing your energy body as described in this chapter and also in chapter titled' Supporting aids for Reiki Practice, it will definitely do you more good.

❑

18
SCIENCE OF MEDITATION

Concentration was just fixing the mind; but meditation is allowing one idea to flow, continuously. Hence, Meditation is an unbroken flow of knowledge of the object on which one meditates. A person, who meditates, at least, half an hour, daily, will be able to face the battle of life with peace and spiritual strength. Meditation kills all pains, suffering and sorrow. It is the most powerful mental and nervine tonic. The divine energy flows freely into, an aspirant during meditation and puts up a benign, soothing influence on the mind, sense-organs and nerves. Thus, the whole body gets rejuvenated. Meditation is the key to unlock the secrets of life, to open the doors of intuitive knowledge and realms to eternal bliss. For meditation, one has to cultivate burning dispassion, burning aspiration or an intense longing for self-realisation. Meditation cannot be attained in a short while. One will have to struggle hard for a long time, be vigilant, diligent and persevering, with a lot of patience. All doubts are cleared, on its own, gradually. A mysterious inner voice will guide you. The best time for Meditation is early morning, between 4 and 6 a.m.

In the beginning, the mind will need a concrete object for meditation. For that, take the form of your master or God and meditate on all the good attributes, such as, omnipotence, perfection, purity, freedom, absolute knowledge, etc.. Later, practise meditation on abstract things, like, effluence of the sun, splendour of the moon, twinkle of the stars, magnificence of the ocean, with its infinite nature. Then, slowly go a step forward and compare these abstract things with your own self. Finally, compare the ocean to the infinite self-consciousness-bliss-knowledge-existence, and the waves, foams and icebergs to the various names and forms of the world. Gaze on the mountains, rivers, the formless air and the all-pervading ether. This will lead you to the realisation of the nameless and formless Soul. This stage of meditation is explained below:

"Meditation is the state of mind, in which it is free of object-perception.

According to this settlement, dhyana means diverting the mind from worldly objects and trying to concentrate it on the self. To concentrate on the self is samadhi.

Having attained dharana, there occurs a continuous flow of perceptive knowledge of the Goal of the meditation which is called meditation. In that state of samadhi the aspirant acquires the fruit of meditation and experiences his own trueself, i.e., Absolute existence–consciousness–bliss as the only reality.

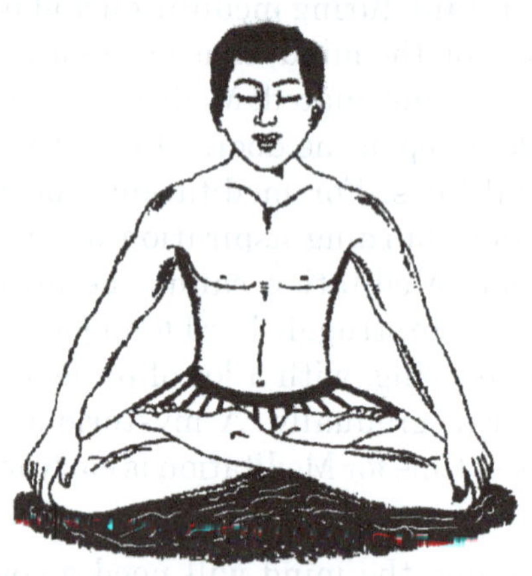

Meditation

Following are the possible obstacles in meditation and the process of removing them is given below:

(*a*) **Sleep and laziness:** Eat less, keep the spine straight, increase the duration of pranayama. It is also good to have a stroll after food.

(*b*) **Overwork and tension:** Avoid unnecessary work, share work with others, work regularly and in a planned manner and leave some things, to be worked out by God.

(*c*) **Misuse of time, things, people, etc:** Remain careful, use everything with care and caution.

(*d*) **Too much indulgence in pleasures:** Reflect on the uselessness of pleasures and try to become detached from them.

(*e*) **Bad company and greed:** Best, if avoided.

(*f*) **Basic passions:** Acting passionless and with discrimination.

(g) **Tension:** Practise relaxation asanas, have good thoughts, help others without any wish, meditate for a fixed period, daily, at the same time, worship the Lord and visit temples.

(*h*) **Criticising others and fault-finding:** Be forgiving and be patient with others, try to remain silent and ignore faults in others.

(*i*) **Unhealthy body:** Practise asanas, pranayama and satkarmas.

(*j*) **Obstacles and lack of-progress:** Have patience and balance of mind.

(*k*) Some other obstacles are tossing of mind (viksepa), rising of latent desires, lack of celibacy, spiritual pride, diseases. For these to be overridden intensive japa-yoga, prarthanfi, trataka are essential. You have to destroy desires through dispassion, discrimination and study of spiritual books. Shun the company of worldly things. Practise celibacy. Give up pride and utilise all necessary means to eradicate diseases, that have come up due to past birth's actions.

(*l*) The greatest obstacle in meditation is when the aspirant tastes the bliss of the lower stages of samadhi (contemplation) and thinks that he has attained liberation. For this, self-analysis and introspection are necessary, as this will save from such a blunder.

Following are some methods of entering into meditation which have been presented, here, keeping in mind the preliminary aspirants as well as the highest level of aspirants, i.e., adepts.

Dainandini Dhyana

At night, before going to sleep, sit in any meditative pose and, then, close the eyes and concentrate on the cidakasa. Then, bring to mind all the major and important events of the day, right from the time of waking up to getting into bed. Also review your actions. Take a pledge not to repeat your mistakes and to perform right actions, even better, in the future. For example, one should take a vow not to be angry, greedy, infatuated, jealous, false, deceptive, etc. Also, pledge to say sorry to others for wrongs, done to them, and try to rectify, wrongs done by you. If necessary, try to remain in silence for some time for atoning all your mistakes. This is repentation. Concentrate on good actions and be determined to remove your faults like anger, greed, etc.

Then, in the morning, after having a bath for practising the daily Yoga routine, sit in some meditative pose and write down the schedule for the day in a copy, mentally. Concentrate on the order, in which the various tasks are to be done and fix a time for each. Repeat the vows taken in the previous night. During the day, perform the tasks in the decided order and in a proper manner.

You shall be very much surprised to see that in a few days you shall be able to succeed in every task undertaken and your daily routine shall be tension-free, calm and peaceful. When this happens your mind shall be better prepared for meditation.

Vigara Dhyana

(Concentration on the thoughts)

We have dealt with this topic in the chapter under the heading antarmauna. This is the second step in the process of entering into meditation. The only difference is now you are not imagining but you are only a witness of all that comes in front of you during the practice.

Mantra Dhyana

(Sylable Meditation)

This topic, too, has been covered in the chapter under the topics japa-yoga and ajapa-japa. This is the third step in the process of meditation. The only difference is now you will not be chanting even mentally but visualising as a witness the mantra's subtle form and meditating on its resonance.

Svasa Dhyana

(Concentration on Breathing)

After the first three steps, i.e., concentration on daily routine, concentration on thoughts and mantra yoga, try to concentrate on the breathing. Close the eyes and let the breathing be, deep. Do not stress too much. Peacefully, concentrate on the exhalation and inhalation. Remain still like a witness. Remain conscious of the pace and volume of breathing. Concentrate on the nostril, being used for breathing - the right, left or both, i.e., ida, pingala or susumna. After a few days of practice, try to notice how the breath is going in and coming out of the nostrils-from the centre of the nostril, from its lower part, upper part, right side or the left side. From the pace of breathing, one shall have to know which element-earth, water, fire, air or ether-is being transmitted.

Untill you have an experience of all this and you have attained control over all the methods of breathing, keep practising.

Sahaja Dhyana

(Natural Meditation)

Sit in any meditative pose and close the eyes and concentrate on the breathing, as much as you can. Then, start chanting OM. For some time, practise ajapa-japa. Thereafter, concentrate the inner vision on the third eye and think of your natural self. In other words, concentrate on your pacific, unified, pure divine joylike-form of true knowledge. Contemplate, thus-I am not the doer or a pleasure-seeker. Happiness-sorrow, jealousy-anger, gain-loss, victory-defeat, fame-ill fame, respect-disrespect, hot-cold and hunger-thirst all are the feelings of the mind. I am beyond all these. I am just a witness. I am the pure Brahman. I am the immortal Soul. Only, the physical body and the mind are affected by birth and death, sleep and awakened state, old age, ailments, smell, touch, beauty and words. These don't affect my true form. Hence, I am free of all boundaries of time, space and place. This is my real form.

Try to concentrate the mind on such thoughts and, then, chant the mantra OM and get up after chanting the shanti-patha, i.e., prayer.

Nada Dhyana

(Meditation of Subtle Sound)

Literally, nada means sound or resonance. But, actually, nada means the flow of consciousness. Consciousness passes through seven states before it is perceived by the senses.

The first state is the formless, pure Brahman, which is the Divine Consciousness - the basis of the other six states of nada.

The second state is OM which has three sub-forms - first is nada, second Bindu and the third kala. Nada is that state of OM in which the subject and the predicate are indistinguishable nonseparate and are present in the dormant form of ignorance. This form is called saguna nirakara, a formless one, but with attributes.

In aggregate, i.e., in macrocosm, superior or universal consciousness, this form is called Tavara or God and in isolation, i.e., microcosm, individual or empirical consciousness, it is called prajna.

The third state is that of bindu. In it, subject and predicate are still indistinguishable but their form is subtle. This is called saguna sakara saksma, a subtle thing, with form and attributes. In aggregate, i.e., macrocosm, superior or universal consciousness it is called antaryami (hiranyagarbha) and in isolation, i.e., microcosm, individual or empirical consciousness, it is called taijasa.

The fourth state of ork is kala. This is the gross form of in aggregate, i.e., macrocosm, superior or universal consciousness, it is called virata and in isolation, i.e., microcosm, individual or empirical consciousness, it is called visva.

The fifth state is that of pard. It is the silent form of the sound. It is also the basic form, which is present in each person's heart, through which the mind knows the word, which is later expressed outside.

The sixth state is pagyanti. The mind "hears" it but the ears cannot. Like a dream, it is a subtle form of sound. At this stage, sound gets a mental form.

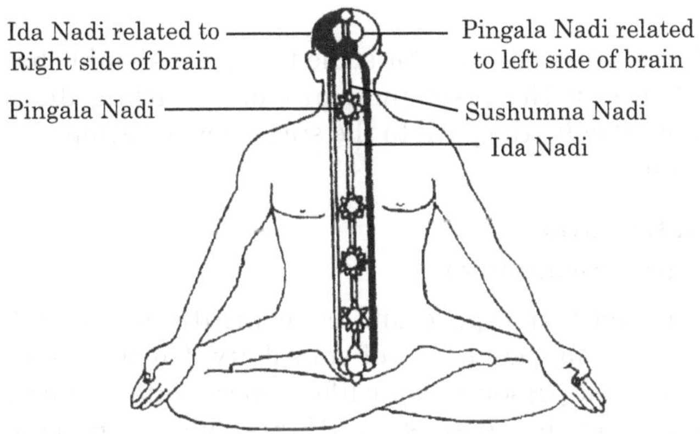

Three Major Nadis

The seventh state is that of madhyama, which is obvious to the mind but not to the senses. Like the period between the state of sleep and awakeness, it lies between the gross and the subtle. It can be heard by the ear as a whispering sound but is not expressed out. Thus, by this a person gains knowledge of the meaning of the sound for himself.

The eighth state is vaikharr. It represents the words that are, spoken. This is the gross form of sound, heard by all.

Hence, the basis of nada-dhydna is the sound in the form of Brahman as stated in the ancient text Mandukyopanisad. In the-dhyana, one concentrates on the beginning of practice of nada sounds of various Indian classical musical instruments. The sounds produced from these instruments, when they are played according to classical music, activate the various chakras of the body. Hence, in the company or under the guidance of the 'guru' (master), one can gain the capability of concentrating on the sound, and thus, attain the union of the soul with the Supreme.

In the absence of a capable guru (master), one could concentrate on the music produced on a flute or a vina. After that, one could sit in some meditative pose with closed eyes. One should shut the ears with cotton or the fingers or in some other manner so that no outside noise disturbs you. Now, one should concentrate on the inner resonance or, whatever sound, one hears within.

After practising thus, for some time, one should chant, and concentrate on the resonance, produced within, due to this chanting. Slowly, the path to the state of meditation shall open up for you.

Bhava Dhyana

(Qualitative Meditation)

Sit in a meditative pose and concentrate on the cidakasa. Contemplate on the virtues of your deity, Guru or some other highly revered person in your life. Concentrate on virtues like kindness, joy, forgiveness, patience, peace, fearlessness, compassion and courage. If necessary, recall some incident or event that brought out that virtue of that person and to which you were a witness. No doubt, these virtues would be completely opposite of your own weaknesses but the thoughts of such virtues would give rise to similar virtues in you.

Bhavatita Dhyana

(Transcendental Meditation)

Sit in some meditative pose for some moments with the eyes closed and remain completely silent. Be a witness and try to concentrate on the thoughts that are rising in your mind. Try to see if there are any thoughts and what they are about. Do not get involved with the thoughts. Just be a witness. Remain aware and repeat over and over again-I am not a part of the play. I am a witness. I am not the thinker. I am just a witness to my thoughts. I am the pure consciousness that is I am Brahman.

Slowly, concentrate on the sacred, pure and divine light-like Soul in between the gap between two consecutive thoughts. Chant oth. With the sound of concentrate on the breathing and the prana, that is moving up and down, the susumna channel.

Feel the resonance of oth, all around. Feel yourself being dissipated, all around, in the form of divine light, along with the resonance of oil. Visualise the universe, present in the divine light, the earth in its place in the universe, your place on earth and your own physical body. Visualise yourself separate from all these as the omnipresent divine element that instills consciousness in everything. Keep concentrating on the sound of oil. When you have practised for some time, visualise the omnipresent divine element returning to the physical body. Concentrate on the divine consciousness in each part of the body and your breathing. Get up after santi-patha, the prayer.

Unmani Kriya

Sit in some meditative pose and practise five rounds of kapalabhoti pranayama. Perform along with the three bandhas and, then, do not open the eyes. But practise ujjayi pranayama. Concentrate on the flow of pranic energy from the muladhara to the chakra and back, even as you chant oth. Imagine that the sound O starts from the difla chakra and, as it reaches the muladhara, it culminates into. Repeat fifty times and, then, chant soham. Rest after every 16 chantings. Chant the soham mantra 52 times, too. Again, repeat with oil. Thereafter, sit peacefully, for some time, and experience the rise of joy and happiness within, due to the just-practised meditation. Do not fall asleep or practise for the sake of entertainment. Return to the normal state and open the eyes after santi-patha prayer.

❑

19
FACTS RELATED TO MEDITATION

Some important facts relating to meditation are as follows:

1. First of all, meditation is not anything that can be forced. Just as sleep comes, naturally, and one cannot go to sleep by one's will, similarly, meditation happens on its own. Still, one has to prepare a bed, bed cover, pillow, blanket, etc., for going to sleep. Similarly, one has to practise the above practices to prepare the mind for meditation. In fact, meditation is an experience that is beyond words just like sleep and the taste of sweets. It can be known only through experience.
2. Meditation has been described as the thoughtless state of mind, self-analysis, conscious analysis of the self, becoming still in the state of mindlessness and so on. But, actually, meditation cannot be described in words.
3. Until one has not become detached from the means of comfort in the material world one cannot dive within and meditate.
4. Actually, the mind is both a boon and a bane for humans. It is through the mind that one can become free of all bonds or get caught in the mire of this world. Hence, one has to practise meditation till order to make the mind, devoted to achieve the goal of spiritual emanciation. The ancient texts state-*mana eva karanam bandhamoksayoh.* Mind is the root cause of bondage and liberation, both.

5. Meditation is a very practical activity. There is no need for any laboratory for it. The body itself is a laboratory in which the mind and the senses are the devices. The science of turning the mind (which always tends to wander outwards) inwards and transcending it above everything can be called as meditation.
6. Through meditation only the sattva, i.e., alpha waves, the most pure among, the four waves produced by the brain (alpha, beta, theta and delta, i.e., sattva, raja, tamah and migra), are generated. As a result, one feels divine joy and peace.
7. The aim of meditation is to concentrate the restless mind.

Benefits of Meditation

The final aim of meditation might or might not be realisation of the Soul but the following benefits surely accrue to a practitioner of meditation:

(*a*) One gains a tension-free mind. The mind becomes still and the body relaxed and peaceful.

(*b*) The mind is not troubled by worldly tensions because the mind, the senses and the experiences, attained through them with the divine Powers, are under control of the yogi.

(*c*) *Yogah karmasu kaugalam*–i.e., according to this verse, through meditation and Yoga, one gains the capability of performing action with wisdom as well as concentration.

(*d*) All the chemical processes and organs of the body, start working flawlessly.

(*e*) Problems like high blood pressure, heart ailments, mental disturbance, tension, sleeplessness, nervous disorders are cured.

❑

20
JAPA-YOGA (SCIENCE OF CHANTING)

This is the best means of purification of the mind. Although it is harder than *prarthana* (prayer), yet, if done with *tapasy* (penance), it proves quick in producing result. Japa means repeating a powerful spiritual word. Repeating a particular word in the mind for progress on the path of attaining oneness with the Supreme Being or Brahman (the all-pervading self) is called japa-yoga. For this, two things are important-the mantra, to be chanted and the mala i.e., rosary, to keep count of the chantings.

Mantra, a syllable, is not an ordinary word or group of words. Rather, it is extraordinary and, through its resonance, the deeprooted tendencies and passions are banished. Mantra is a group of words instilled with the powers of some. Hence, it is better to get a mantra from a 'guru' (master). The best mantra for an aspirant is one which is in perfect harmony with his soul and which awakens devotion in him. There are infinite mantras, pertaining to the different gods, goddesses and deities in different religions and sects. Hence, it is best to ask the 'guru' which mantra would suit one and, then, one should get 'diksha' (spiritual initiation in a particular mantra-practice) from the 'guru.'

A mala i.e., rosary has 108 beads. Each bead is secured with a knot which represents the worldly bonds and is called brahmagranthi. Other than the 108 beads, there is one more, which is tied separately, to the main string of the rosary. It is called sumeru. It helps in keeping a tab on the number of rounds of the rosary. There are rosaries with 11, 21, 27, 33, 36 and 54 beads for special purposes. Rosaries, with beads of rudraksa (seed of a sacred tree), sphatika (rock-crystal), etc., are used for different purposes.

There can be four types of japa–likhita (written), vaikhari (oral), upaihgu (murmuring) and manasika (mental). Those with a very fickle and restless mind should practice likhita japa. To write the mantra in beautiful handwriting on a page with a feeling of devotion and love for one's deity is called likhita japa. When, through this type of japa, the senses become calm and concentrated, then, one should start vaikhari japa. In vaikhari japa, one should sit in a meditative pose and relax the mind and the body. Then, one should close the eyes and forming the image of the deity in one's mind, one should chant the mantra, clearly and loudly. But this should be practised alone in the room. One should concentrate on the resonance of the mantra. This is called vaikhari japa.

Then, seated as before, if one chants the mantra silently, murmuring in such a way that the mantra can be heard only by himself and not even by a person sitting beside, is called upanshu japa. Silent chanting does not mean that one can get away with incorrect pronunciation. Rather, it means that if someone else is in the room he or she should be able to see your lips moving but not hear the mantra. The last is manasika japa. In it, one is to sit as before but one should chant the mantra in the mind without even moving the lips or tongue and keeping the mouth shut. This is the best method of chanting.

The preliminary aspirants should practise likhita japa. A little advanced category of aspirants could practise the other three types. (1) those capable of only vaikhari japa; (2) those capable of both vaikhari and upanshu japas; and (3) those who chant one round of vaikhari, two rounds upaighu and three rounds manasika. The highest category of aspirants, i.e., adepts for elephant practise only manasika japa.

By chanting a mantra daily right from the day one, you get it from the Master, unto the time of death, is called nitya japa, eternal or obligatory chant. Chanting a certain number in a certain period of days, as directed by the mantra, is called anusthana. The highest form of anusthana is called purascarana, which is quite tough.

Rules for the Chanting of Mantras

- The rosary should not be seen by others. Hence, it should be held in the hand, inside a cloth pouch, called gomukhi.
- One should not cross the sumeru the 109th bead, when moving the beads.
- One should not touch the forefinger and.the little finger to the rosary.
- Pronunciation of the mantra should be clear and correct.
- The speed of chanting should be constant so that it is in rhythm.
- Chanting should be done without any desire.
- Do not reveal the mantra to anyone.
- One should choose a particular spot, a particular sitting posture, a particular cotton or woollen piece of cloth or blanket and a particular time, daily, for the chanting.
- It is more effective to chant the mantra, facing the north or east.
- Keep concentrating on the meaning of the mantra and the deity, whom one is worshipping while chanting the mantra. It is said in the text Patanjali Yoga-Sutra (1/27).

The mind is clouded by three obstacles on the path of Yoga restlessness, impurity and foolishness. The aim of japa is to free the mind of these three. When the mind is pure, then, it becomes capable of realising the soul.

Ajapa –Japa (Non-stop eternal chanting)

To keep repeating the mantra is called japa. The japa becomes ajapa, when the mantra gets repeated in the mind on its Ajapa-japa goes on, subconsciously, all the time, while japa is consciously.

Ajapa-japa is a complete sadhana (spiritual practice) in it. If this starts and one becomes aware of it, then, one can very enter into the state of meditation, i.e., dhyana. This type of helps in banishing passions, desires and fears and makes the very pure.

When there is an explosion of the latent passion tendencies, one should not react. Rather, one should just watch them like an audience. Otherwise, these passions can lead to spiritual downfall. This type of japa also frees the mind and body of all ailments and weaknesses.

Generally, "soham" mantra is used for this purpose, but other mantra also can be used.

In the beginning, i.e., first stage, the aspirant should concentrate on the breathing. He should practise this meditative pose. Breathe in and feel the chest and abdomen region,becoming empty. After concentrating on the breath for sometime, in the second stage, feel the resonance of the same, while inhaling, and, ham, when exhaling. Do this for breath. After one month of practice, reverse the process.

In second stage, first breathe out and feel the resonance ham and, then, breathing in, and feel the resonance of so. In words, in the second stage, chant hamso.

In the third stage, chant so hamso.

In the fourth stage, continuously, chant mentally only a soham so that there is no break between so and ham.

Pratyahara

In the fifth stage, chant, mentally, performing khechari-mudra and ujjayi pranayama.

In the sixth stage, move the conscience on the chakras of the kundalini. If possible, continue to be aware of the resonance and try to concentrate the prana on each chakra. In the last stage, one becomes a witness to what was happening in the earlier stages. One has to be fully conscious, in this stage, and not fall asleep.

When a person is able to continue in the final stage he enters into the highest level of meditation and, then, into samadhi.

Precautions and Guidelines

Practise withdrawal of senses, one by one, beginning with the most turbulent one and this has to be done, gently not vehemently. Detach your mind from its desired objects. The best way is to withdraw the senses, too, along with prana, which is the cause of action. You have to be alert and vigilant in annihilating all desires with the sword of dispassion and the axe of discrimination. For this, one cannot do on one's accord, so guru and God's grace are essential. For that, devotion and surrender are the tools.

Observance of silence, moderation in diet, steadiness in pose, dispassion, regularity in the practice of asana and pranayama, patience, contentment, perseverance, tenacity, celibacy, seclusion, discrimination between the real and the non-real are all aids to pratyahara.

The obstacles to pratyahara are passions and desires, too much working, too much mixing with worldly people, too much worldly activity, too much food, too much walking, too much curiosity in external affairs, slackness and laziness in practices, etc. Every practitioner should be careful about one's own wavery mind and recognise by self-analysis which quality is dominant in him. Accordingly, one has to decide the practices that he has to adopt and way of life that he has to lead to attain salvation, at the earliest.

❑

21
ANTAH DARSANA (INNER VISUALISATION)

In antah darsana (the inner visualisation), one has to visualise all the events and actions, that took place outside, in day or night time in the mind, like a dream. But one should not fall asleep and one should be aware that this witnessing is not actually a dream but a conscious effort. In this practice, one has to recall and visualise all the important events and actions, involved in it, right from the time of waking up, in the morning to the time of lying down to sleep.

You have to visualise exactly all details like going to a friend's place, the exact location of his house, the vehicle you used and the people you saw. Or, you could recall going to the temple, the priest, who greeted you, the various utensils kept there, the ritual performed there, the worship you performed and the *prasada* (sweets offered to the Gods), that you got. If you travelled, then, recall the bus or the train you used, the things you saw on the way, the various stations or stops that came on the way and the hustle and bustle, there. You could also recall natural scenes and events, the stars, the sun, the moon which you saw or the different colours and shapes, that you witnessed. If a student, one could recall the scene of one's college or school, one's class, the teacher teaching the class, etc.

In the final stage of this practice, one should pronounce the names of the objects and persons, mentally, that one recalls. This practice increases one's memory and prepares one for further practice.

Cidakasa Darsana

(Cerebral or Conscious Visualisation)

The dark and black space that one visualises in the place of the third eye, i.e., the eyebrow centre, when one closes the eyes is called cidakas. Concentrating the mind on this spot and, then, visualising the following types of scenes is called cidakasa darsana.

Sit in a meditative pose. Close the eyes and position the hands in dhyan-mudra. Concentrate on the sounds around you. Then visualise your own body in the mind. Visualise your physical form seated on the floor. Concentrate the mind on the breathing. Then, concentrate it on the cidakasa. It has no shape, but if one continues to concentrate, then, after some time, different colours start to appear. Keep viewing them. Now visualise this dark space, not just on the third eye, but all around you, everywhere. One can pronounce the names of the colours one is seeing, mentally. Now, visualise your own form but with a divine radiance in the cidakas. Concentrate on the sound of OM, emanating from there. Keep viewing the images that might appear. When ending the practice, perform the reverse, i.e., first, concentrate on the breathing, then, the body and, lastly, on the sounds all around. Then, get up.

Antarmauna

(Inner Silence)

Mauna means to be silent outside and inside. In order to reach this state, one shall have to cut oneself off from the commotion outside and restlessness of the mind and the senses. In this practice, a person has an experience of being a witness to everything, which is very important for meditation.

Antarmauna can be divided into three stages–(1) vak-sathyama (control of speech); (2) vatig-mauna (silence of speech); and (3) antarmauna (silence of mind, too).

The first stage of antarmauna is called vak-sathyama (control of speech). The eyes, ears and the tongue destroy the peace of the mind and make it tense and worried. Among these three–

speech creates most disturbances. Hence, if the speech is controlled, the rest two are controlled on their own. For the practice of vaksathyama, one has to get into the habit of speaking less. For this, remember the following tips–do not stress your point too much speak after due thought, do not get into an argument, do not get involved in criticising others, do not get perturbed by adverse circumstances, do not speak anything that might hurt anyone and, finally, keep your words and voice sweet. Hence, vak-salhyama means to speak for the good of others, keeping their respect and feelings in mind.

The second stage of antarmauna is vatig-mauna (silence of speech). The ancient texts state–*maunum sarvdrtha sadhanam* (silence is the best way of attaining all wishes). Complete rest of the tongue is called vafig-mauna. When a person is totally silent, the voice of the Lord becomes obvious. This practice increases power of thought, memory and intelligence. Such a person can, then, read the mind of others. Through complete silence, one can know about the restlessness of the mind, the hidden evil tendencies and one's passions. Then, it becomes easy to control them and transform the mind, completely, through the practices, suggested in the ancient texts. An aspirant gains knowledge, divine power and several virtues, like the capability of solving all problems, influencing others through one's speech, etc., because the divine voice works and not his selfish voice.

The third stage of antarmauna can be divided into five substages.

In the first stage, one has to remain aware of the events and the sounds, outside. One should hear and see everything but not react. One has to remain a mere silent witness.

In the second stage, one has to curb the tendency of the eyes and ears to be directed outwards into external objects, i.e., one has to close the eyes and ears and concentrate on the mind, on the thoughts, on its reactions and the various images, being generated in it. Do witness all this but be aware of the self. Be like a witness and do not get involved in the thoughts or the scenario.

In the third stage, go through the first and the second stages, alternatively. In other words, practise outer and inner awareness.

In the fourth stage, sit in a peaceful and isolated place, generate images in the mind and witness them. This practice is called manoraj. These are of two types–natural and artificial. The former is to be avoided and the latter has to be practised. Generally, manorajya is said to be an obstacle on the way to meditation and samadhi, because, in it, a person loses his awareness and becomes completely engrossed and wastes his time. This is natural manorajya here, i.e., in fourth stage too the person does create images in the mind and witnesses them but he does not get involved in them. This is artificial manoriya. In natural manoriya, the aspirant does not create images but, whenever the mind wishes, due to passions, starts to imagine things, he should be aware of it and not get engrossed into it. For this, the aspirant will have to be alert, all the 24 hrs. This is very difficult. Previously, it was mentioned that the former is to be avoided. But, if an adept can practice, being alert all the 24 hrs, then, it is not harmful. Such an aspirant gains a capability to curb unnecessary imaginations and be able to utilise the mind's energy, properly and positively. Hence, here, it proves helpful rather than be an obstacle.

In the fifth stage, the mind has to be made totally calm. One has to concentrate on the divine conscience, that is formless. One has to concentrate on divine light. This is a state of stunned silence for the mind. It is like unconsciousness. The difference is that, in unconsciousness, the person is not aware of anything but, here, the person is aware of the state of total silence and also experiences the all-pervading consciousness-existence-bliss.

When the aspirant has perfected this practice, his mind becomes prepared for meditation. Up to now the different techniques were discussed as per the Himalayan tradition. Now, let us see the different techniques as adopted by my master's tradition.

The key to dharana is that, first, you have to recognise your mind, i.e., decide the quality of your mind, then, accordingly, you can choose the object of concentration. Once you start on anything, then you have to avoid the mental confrontation, that will increase the ability of concentration. Relaxation and concentration are interrelated. Therefore, before starting practice perform some relaxation postures, little pranayama, yoga-nidra (little), prarthana and trataka besides niskama karma yoga and yuktahara. Training of mind, systematically, is very much necessary for transformation of consciousness. Training of mind constitutes three steps. Firstly, concept of dharana should be clear, secondly, intensity of experience and, finally, intensity of concentration. To make the second step successful, you have to practise inner visualisation. But during this process, one will have to face many obstacles. They are as follows:

1. Visions–both good, like, angels, demi-gods, etc., and bad like snakes, lions, devils, etc., come up. If you are able to remain calm and unaffected, then, your practice is proceeding unimpeded.
2. Kundalini awakening–a person, in whom partial awakening of kundalini has occurred, a susumna channel has not been aroused, dharana is impossible. For this pranayama perfection is essential.
3. Sensitiveness sensual and emotional feelings develop in the lower centres, forcing you into the external world, because purification of prana and psychic centres increases the production of sexual fluid; for this, celebacy has to be maintained and sexual energy has to be transformed under the guidence of an expert master.
4. Encountering illness.
5. Disillusion.
6. Changing practices.
7. Applying short-cuts.
8. Excessive social activities.
9. Irregular diet.
10. Imbalanced diet.
11. Unnecessary tensions.

Once you are capable of overcoming obstacles and you have trained your mind, you can practise the different techniques of dharana, mentioned in Yoga, Tantra and Upanisads. Some have already been discussed. The rest will be dealt with briefly, now.

The techniques are as follows, which are to be done under the guidance of an expert master.

Yogic and Tantric Dharana

1. Kaya-sthairyam – Body stability.
2. Chakra suddhi – Purification of psychic centres.
3. Ajapa-japa – Done in 10 stages.
   - one – Frontal passage rotation.
   - two – Spinal passage rotation.
   - three – Frontal passage rotation with ujjayi.
   - four – Spinal passage rotation with ujjayi.
   - five – Arohana-avarohana rotation.
   - six – Ida-pingala elliptical rotation.
   - seven – Pingala-ida elliptical rotation.
   - eight – Ida-pingala spinal rotation.
   - nine – Pingala-ida spinal rotation.
   - ten – Opening the chakras.
4. Trataka – Done in 4 stages.
   - one – external concentration.
   - two – external–internal concentration.
   - three – internal concentration.
   - four – void concentration.

Upanisadic Dharana

1. External ether concentration.
2. Internal ether concentration.
3. Cerebral ether concentration.
4. Hearty ether concentration.
5. Little ether concentration.
6. Miscellaneous concentrations.

one	–	Five elements concentrations.
two	–	Chakras concentration.
three	–	Five sheaths concentration.
four	–	Five prana concentration.

7. Destructivity concentration.
8. The five concentration together.

❑

22
KNOW YOUR CHAKRAS

Everythig is energy. You can facilitate the entrance of energy into your body through the top of your head. Here is one way to start learning how to consciously absorb the life force.

Sit quietly and close your eyes. Imagine warm white or blue light glowing about six inches above the top of your head. Open your head to receive the light, which flows down your legs, down your arms, and out of you. Then become filled to overflowing simply by closing your fingers and toes so the chi builds inside you. Become saturated, even to the outside of your aura, the field of energy that surrounds every organism. Become replete with energy. Take your time. Then let the light grow until it surrounds you. Notice how you feel. When you are ready open your eyes. The protection of the light will remain with you.

Chakras: Spinning Energy Wheels

For thousands of years, Eastern philosophers have believed that the human organism gets most of its energy from invisible waves or rays entering through the top of the head. Every parent knows the soft spot on a baby's head, the fontanelle, must be protected for the child's first months of life. The bones of the skull naturally close this opening with age, to protect the delicate brain tissues. Just as this opening is though to have received energy from the mother while she holds her child in the womb. Eastern tradition teaches that the crown of the head remains the primary entrance place of vital chi throughout life. In addition, significant amounts of chi also come up through the spine and through the feet, from Mother Earth.

As the life force enters the body, it passes through and activates the seven primary chakras. The word chakra means wheel, and is an ancient East Indian symbol, used in this sense to mean a centre of physical and psychic energy. The seven major chakras are known by many different names. We prefer the East Indian terms.

1. Muladhara
2. Svadhisthana
3. Manipura
4. Anahata
5. Vishudha
6. Ajna
7. Sahasrara

Also indicated on the accompanying chakra diagram are two secondary chakras. We like to call the palm chakra (8) by its Chinese name, Lao Kun, and we refer to the chakra in the soles of the feet (9) as Yung Chuan, "Bubbling Spring." We mention these secondary chakras in some of the dynamic meditations, for example, in Red Dragon chi kung, where pyramids are formed between the chakras.

There are, of course, many other energy points and junctions along the energy meridians (which correspond to our nervous system) which lace our bodies. The acupuncturist uses these points to cure illness and relieve pain.

The major chakras are located along the spinal column, and are closely related to the endocrine system, the nervous system, and the circulatory system, all of which influence hormonal secretions in some way. The accompanying illustration shows approximately where the chakras are located, and you can see for yourself how they relate to the diagrams of body systems.

At the peak of health and vitality, our chakras spin or vibrate at great speed. As we grow older or develop unhealthy habits and begin to lose vitality, the rate of vibration of some or all of the chakras slows down. This gradual decrease in vibration affects the flow of hormones released by the endocrine system. Too much, too little-either condition brings on the familiar symptoms of aging, and also increases the possibility of disease.

Your task is to mix and balance the incoming energy, the earth energy, with the energy coming in from the universe, and to create a system of chakras that literally "hums." If balance occurs, each chakra will be open, the physical body will perform optimally, and a unified organism will result.

Are you "In the Pink"?

When concentrating on the different chakra centres of your body, you may see certain colours when your eyes are closed. Once your goals become more spiritual, you may feel drawn toward particular colours, depending on the chakra you are working with. It is all a matter of what feels right to you at each particular stage of your spiritual development.

Rainbow colours are almost universally accepted to represent the chakra centres, although there is not such agreement as to which colour symbolises which chakra. But this does not point to one being right and one being wrong, rather, it points to the difference in what colour was seen by a particular master while in meditation.

The number of light waves that come to our eyes each second is known as the frequency of light. the different frequencies are perceived as different colours. The red end of the light spectrum. or rainbow, is the lowest frequency of light waves. The blue end is the highest frequency.

And, of course, light is not the only thing that has a frequency because it is composed of waves of energy. All parts of the universe, flesh and blood, plant and mineral vibrate because each is a different form of energy. Our chakras are concentrations of energy which seem to have their own integrity and their own separate identity and frequency. You can "Feel" someone behind you without actually hearing, seeing or noticing him or her in any way other than identifying a field of energy that is vibrating a bit differently than your energy body.

We are presenting the colour scheme and key words we are most comfortable with, based on the colours our energy work has shown us. You can adapt it according to what colours you identify with when working with each chakra.

1. **Mooladhara Chakra:** It is located at the base of the spine. It is also called as Root or Base Chakra. Persons with weak Root Chakra tend to be weak and drained of vitality.

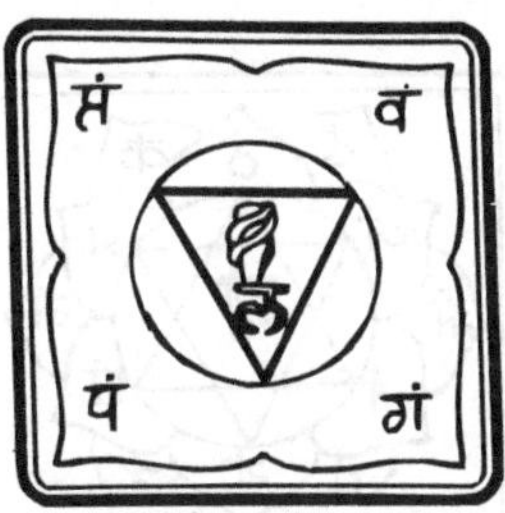

Mooladhara Chakra

2. **Swadhisthana Chakra:** It is located near sacrum or public area and slightly below navel. Due to malfunctioning of this Chakra one can suffer from sex related diseases, high B.P. backache, kidney problems and constipation etc.

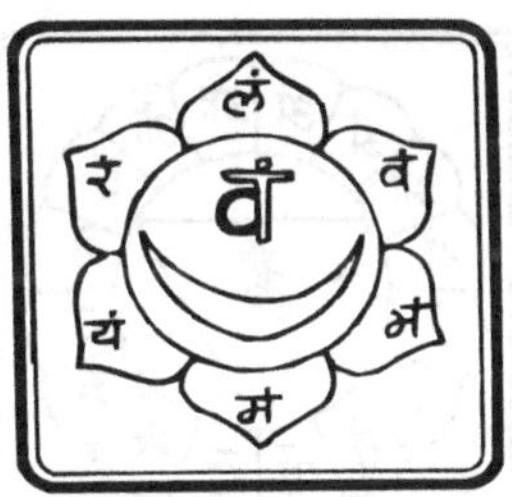

Swadhisthana Chakra

3. **Manipura Chakra:** It is located slightly above the navel and below the ribs. Due to malfunctioning of this Chakra one can suffer from digestive disorders, skin problems, heart problems, asthma etc.

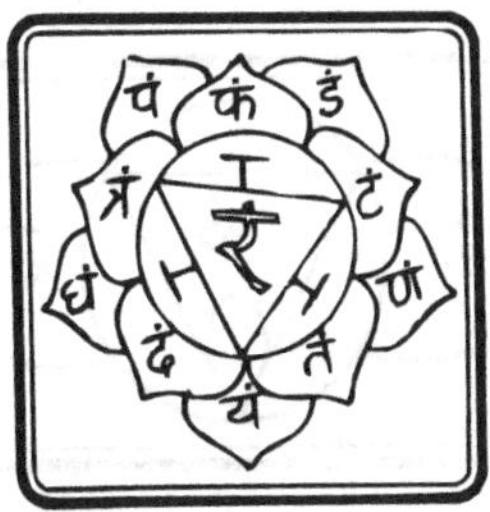

Manipura Chakra

4. **Anahata Chakra:** It is located in the centre of the chest, at the height of the heart. Malfunctioning of this Chakra can cause heart and circulatory ailments, lung ailments and many more problems.

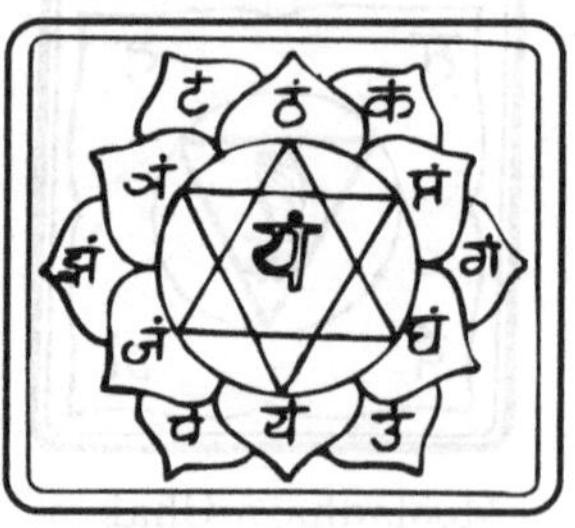

Anahata Chakra

5. **Vishuddha Chakra:** It is located in the hollow of the throat. Due to malfunctioning of this Chakra one can suffer from throat related diseases.

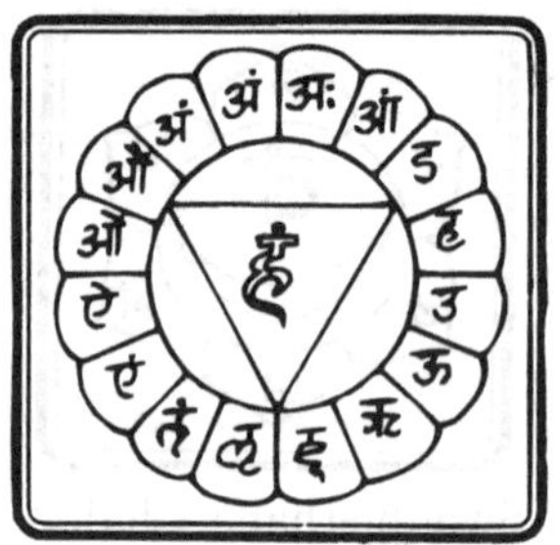

Vishuddha Chakra

6. **Ajna Chakra:** It is located between the eyebrows. Due to te malfunctioning of this Chakra one can suffer from diseases related to endocrine glands, nervous system, sense organs etc.

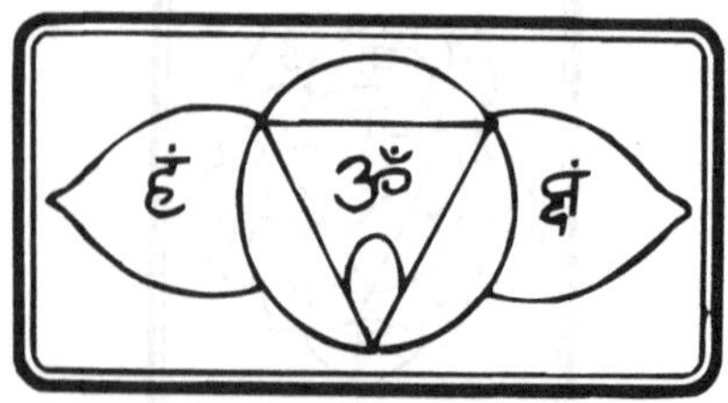

Ajna Chakra

7. **Sahasrar Chakra:** It is located at the top of one's head. Due to malfunctioning of this Chakra one can suffer from diseases related to Pineal gland and the Cerebral cortex.

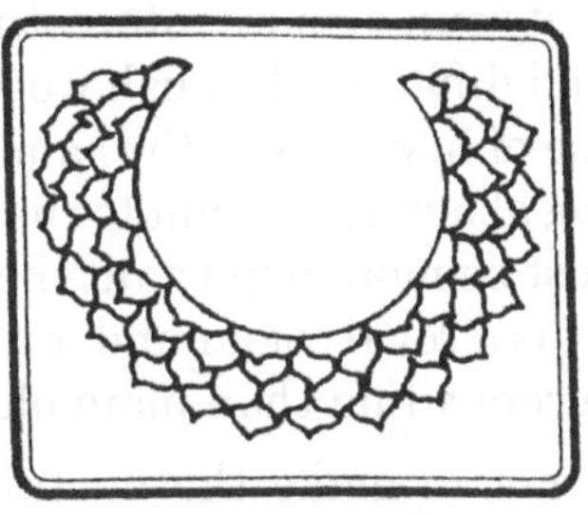

Sahasrar Chakra

Chakra Colours and Keywords Chart I

Muladhara	Red	The base chakra relating to survival and procreation.
Svadhistana	Orange	The health and pleasure chakra relating to well being immunity from disease and pleasure in life.
Manipura	Yellow	The power chakra or solar plexus, relating to a reservoir of spiritual and physical energy which gives strength to all the other chakras and keeps them healthy.
Anahata	Green	The heart chakra, relating to unconditional acceptance which frees the other chakras from ego, melds our heart's love energy with cosmic wisdom, and makes the bridge from physical to spiritual and from known to unknown.
Vishudha	Blue	The throat chakra, relating to creativity and self-expression, the gateway to communication with the unkbown.
Ajna	Violet	The third eye chakra, relating to intution, paranormal powers, and psychic awareness.
Sahasrara	Indigo	The crown chakra, relating to liberation into the cosmic realm,bliss.

Develop Patience

Here in the West, we are competitive and impatient, attributes which do not promote spiritual development. We want to work in the stars because it sounds more interesting, more exciting; it is something new and different. English words tend to give false impressions, because of how we use the same works in everyday life. Without thinking about it, we want to rush on to do "advanced work" because it must be more important than "beginning work" And, of course, violet is a royal colour and must therefore be more deserving of our concentration than plain old red.

It is important not to make the mistake of confusing the terms "higher" and "better." Muladhara, Savadhisthana and Manipura are known as the earth-based chakras. Vishudha, Ajna, and Sahasrara are the cosmic chakra. Right now, most of us are living in the physical plane and our firm foundation, our base, is very well developed. But the earth based chakras all need nourishment and attention. At the same time that you are developing the chakras that are symbolically higher in the body and which deal more with the spiritual aspects of life, give your three lower chakras nourishment. Try not to forget that while we are on the physical plane. Even though our heads may be in the clouds, our feet are still on the ground.

The Cleansing Breath Technique

This is best done in a kneeling position in which you can bend forward freely. Place your hands on your stomach, left hand over right, just underneath your rib cage, Bend forward and gently press out all the air by pulling in with your hands and expelling all the air in your lungs.

Then, take a complete breath in about six or seven good, sized sniffs, going back each time until you are sitting upright on your heels. Your diaphragm will expand downward as your lungs fill, your stomach will push outward, and your rib cage will come up. Don't hold this large breath more than a few seconds. Release it explosively, all at once, through your nose.

Assist the rapid and complete cleansing by pulling in with your hands and by leaning forward as you exhale to get all the air out.

Up to seven cleansing breaths can be done at one sitting. this cleansing breath technique is beneficial to anyone, but especially for those exposed to a polluted environment (which does include most of us.).

The following technique is a breath balance which can be performed before any exercise.

Nadi Sodhana

The purpose of this "breath of union" is for you to begin to breathe equally through both nostrils. It is an effective technique for balancing the energy in your body and the two hemispheres of your brain, to help you attain a more balanced state of awareness.

To begin, sit on the floor, cross-legged if possible or in another comfortable meditation posture. Your left hand, with thumb and index fingers joined, rests on your left knee. The index finger of your right hand rests on your forehead, between your eyebrows at the third eye chakra. The thumb of your right hand will be used to close your right nostril and the middle finger will close your left nostril.

You will probably be breathing through one nostril more than the other. For the purpose of these instructions, we will call the right nostril the dominant one. If you find you are breathing more from the left nostril, begin the breathing sequence in reverse of what we describe, starting out with your left hand closing your nostrils, and so on.

To begin Nadi Sodhana, inhale and press your right nostril (or whichever is your dominant nostril) closed with your right thumb and exhale forcefully through your left nostril. Inhale through your left nostril as you count to seven. Now close your left nostril with your middle finger of your right hand and hold your breath again for a count of seven.

Release your right nostril and exhale through it for a count of seven. Immediately, still keeping your left nostril closed, inhale slowly through your right nostril for a count of seven. Assume Moola bandha as you make this slow inhalation. After you count to seven, close both nostrils and hold your breath for another count of seven. Now release the left nostril and exhale through your left nostril for a count of seven, releasing Moola bandha as you do so.

Repeat the entire sequence seven times in all. Remember, do not hold your breath if you have high blood pressure. You will gain a balancing benefit from this technique.

Chakra Chart II

Sanskrit	English	Body root	Plexus and gland
Muladhara	Root support	Coccyx	Pelvic plexus Testes and ovaries
Swadhisthana	One's own place (Below)	Sacral vert. Navel	Hypogastric plexus Adrenal glands
Manipura	Gem city	Lumbar vert. Navel (above)	Solar plexus pancreas and liver
Anahata	Unstruck Sound	Thoracic vert. Heart region	Cardiac plexus Thymus gland
Vishuddha	Purity centre	Cervical vert. Throat area	Pharyngeal plexus Thyroid gland Parathyroids
Ajan	Command	Nasion between eyes	Nasociliary plexus Pituitary gland
Sahasrara	1,000-petaled	Bregma Top of head	Cerebrum Pineal gland

❑

23
ENERGIZING CHAKRAS

The origin of these exercise is unclear. They were probably developed in Tibet or India and are said to be part of an ancient and secret system of Yoga for physical rejuvenation. When practiced regularly, they do seem to have a powerful influence. Try them for at least a month and see how they work for you.

When you are in optimum health, your chakras spin at a high frequency of vibration. This frequency tends to lower with age and inactivity. When the spin of the chakras slows down, the result is an increasingly unresponsive endocrine system. The flow of hormones to regulate body functions is affected, and often the singals are ignored or misunderstood by other parts of the body. A domino effect begins to occur because the endocrine glands have a close partnership. If one is not working properly, it will influence the others.

The purpose of these exercises is to energize and restore the spin of the chakras to their youthful rate. This is a desirable outcome, because if the chakra system is perfectly balanced, it is said that the body will not age.

Each of the energizers is meant to be repeated 21 times to make a complete set. You should perform all five sets in the morning and then again in the evening, if you wish.

Once you become proficient, you should be able to complete all five energizers in about 10 minutes. But in the beginning, you may have difficulty performing all the energizers perfectly and with this many repetitions.

Do not become impatient with your progress. Do the best you can, and gradually the exercises will become easier. Start by performing each energizer just three times. Increase by adding two or more repetitions with each week of practice. They should be done at a speed comfortable for you, but you should be careful to fully inhale and fully exhale as you do them.

Energizer uses no energy locks. All the rest require that you maintain Moola bandha (root lock) throughout. Let your breathing pattern establish the rhythm.

Energizer 1

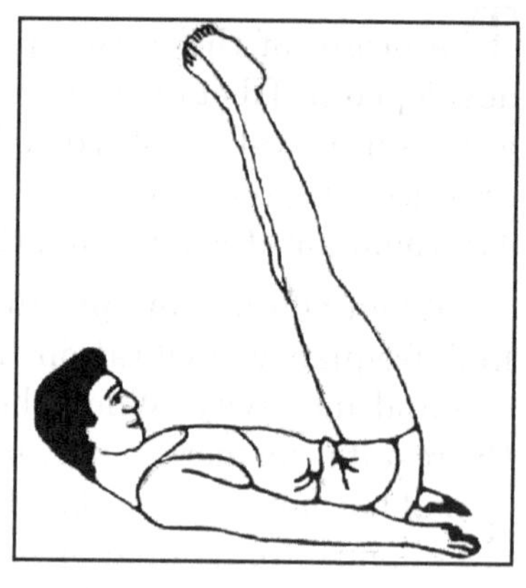

Using no locks, stand erect with your arms outstretched at shoulder level. Your right hand is turned palm up, your left hand is turned palm down. Now apin in a clockwise direction (to your right). Choose something in the room at eye level and count each time you pass it. Spin at a comforable speed until you feel a little dizzy.

Energizer 2

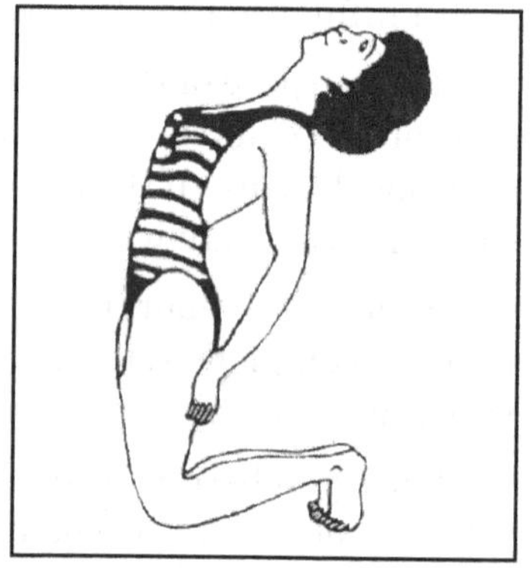

Lie flat on the floor on your back. Your arms should be along your sides, with your palms on the floor. Maintain Moola bandha. Inhale and raise your head off the floor, bringing your chin firmly against your chest. As you raise your head, also lift your legs as high off the floor as possible. Don't let your knees bend. Now, exhale and lower both your head and legs back the floor. Repeat up to 21 times. Remember to breathe in when your head and legs are raised and breathe out as you lower them.

Energizer 3

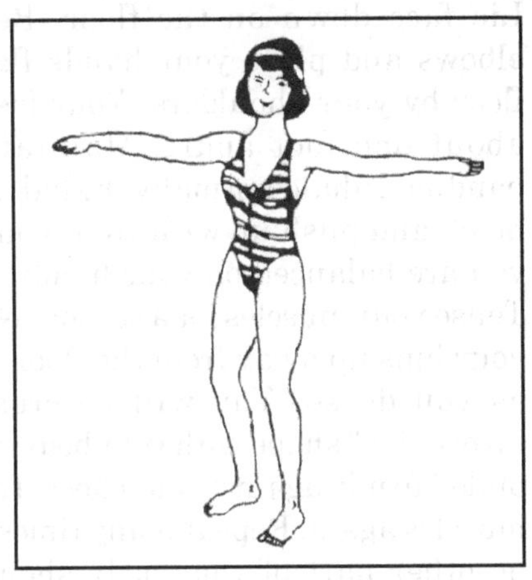

Kneel with your body upright, with your hands behind you against the backs of your thighs. Maintain Moola bandha. Inhale normally. Exhale and lower your head so your chin is pressed firmly against your chest. Then inhale as you vigorously bend your head and neck backward, arching your spine. This should create a stretch from your stomach to your chin. Your hands will act as a brace against your thighs to support the arching movement. Repeat many times.

Energizer 4

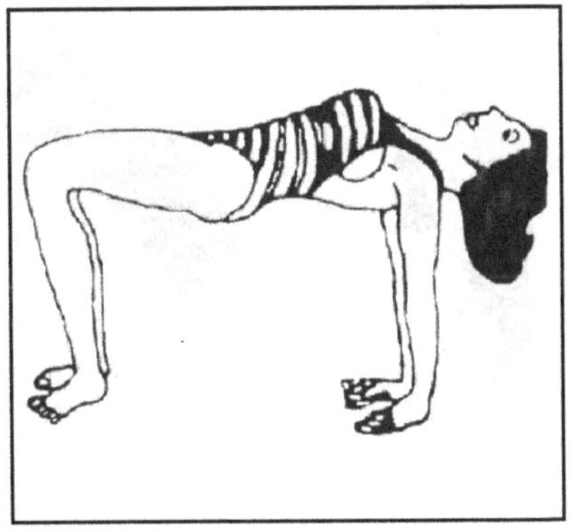

Sit on the floor with your legs straight in front and your feet about 12 inches apart. Your upper body is held erect. The palms of your hands are resting on the floor beside your hips. Maintain Moola bandha. Inhale normally, then exhale and tuck your chin down firmly to your chest. Inhale and toss your head backward as far as it will comfortably go, at the same time raising your body off the floor. Your knees will be bent and your arms will be straight. The trunk of your body will be parallel to the floor while your arms and lower legs will be perpendicular to the floor. Tense your muscles while in this position, then relax and exhale as you return to the sitting position you started with. Repeat this exercise many times.

Energizer 5

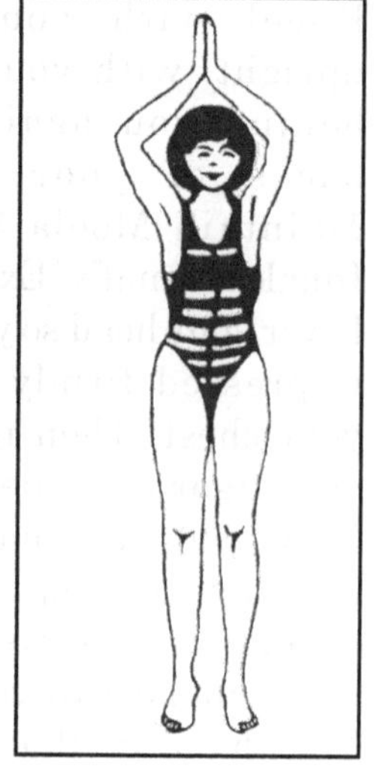

Lie face down on the floor. Bend your elbows and place your hands flat on the floor by your shoulders. Your feet will be about one foot apart. Maintain Moola bandha. Inhale normally. Exhale, lift your head, and push up with your arms so that you are balanced on your hands and toes. Tense your muscles for a second. Now, push your hips up away from the floor, inhaling as you do so. You will be creating an inverted "v" shape with your body, your chin pulled firmly against your chest. Tense your muscles again. Repeat many times. Ideally, no other part of your body should touch the floor except your hands and toes as you flex your body back and forth between the head up position and the inverted 'v.'

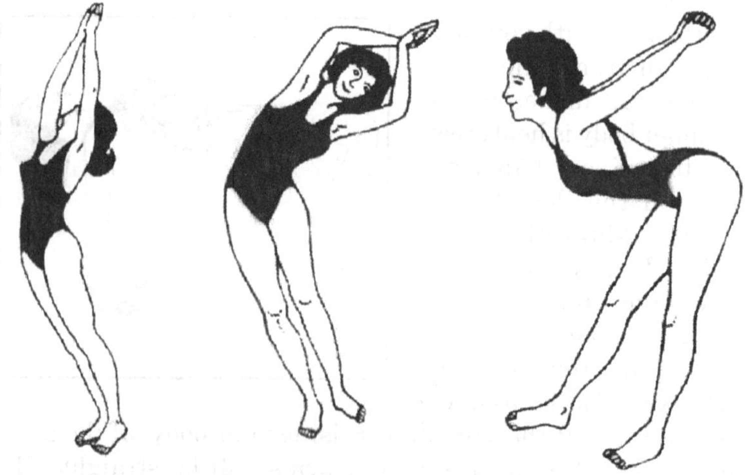

Chakra Energizing

Crane Draws in chi

Standing with slightly bent knees, inhale through your nose as you lift your hands to waist level. Your elbows should be bent and your palms up. Exhale, pushing out to the front with your hands palms facing forward. Inhale and raise your arms up to the cosmos, palms up. Exhale as you bring your hands down. Repeat two more times to complete the circulation of chi.

Energizing in Indian Way

In our western lifestyle, many of us spend the greater part of our waking lives sitting, often hunched over something in front of us. This causes our neck and shoulders to become tense and stiff, and there is no free physical movement or energetic flow. When your muscles are stiff the energy channels become blocked, in turn affecting the organs, glands and nerves into which these channels feed.

The following are isometric exercises from the traditions of East India. They use dynamic tension to energize and relax the body. When you work the muscles against each other isometrically, the tension briefly restricts blood and chi flow. When the tension is relaxed, the muscles receive a rush of oxygen rich blood and chi. This alternation of tension and relaxation of deprivation and replenishment of your bdoy's physical and spiritual life forces, leaves you energized; your muscles will also be much looser than before.

These exercises take so little time and space that they could even be performed on your coffee or lunch break at work. Have your beverage when you pause from working if you wish, but add some isometrics for even more refreshment for your body. These exercises are also an excellent preliminary for any other set of exercises.

Stretching Up Ist Step

Stand relaxed, with your arms at your sides, Inhale and sweep your arms up from your sides until they are over head, at the same time going up on your toes. When your hands reach above your head, press your palms together to create isometric tension in your arms. Hold your breath while in this position for a moment. Take a small sniff of air to allow an even exhalation, then exhale as you lower your arms and come down from your toes. When your hands have just separated but are still facing overhead, rotate your wrists so your palms point away from each other. Continue to lower your arms until they are down to your sides.

Perform the stretch ten times, then relax. This exercise will help open the front of your lungs.

Stretching Up IInd Step

Perform the stretch as in Stretching Up I, except for a different hand position. This time, press the backs of your hands together. Inhale as you go up, press the backs of your hands together, maintain the tension for a few moments, then exhale and come back down. Perform the stretch seven times, then relax.

Sidebends

Stand relaxed, with your arms at your sides. Inhale and stretch your arms overhead, crossing your wrists so that your palms are together. Create tension by pressing your palms together tightly. Exhale as you bend slowly to your right. Inhale as you return to the upright position, your arms still overhead. Repeat until you have done the bend seven times to the right. Recross your hands the other way, and now perform the bend seven times to the left. Maintain the tension at your palms throughout the exercise, then relax with your arms at your sides.

Variation

Use this exercise if your wrists and hands are too stiff for the hand position in Sidebends.

Inhale and stretch your arms overhead, hooking your thumbs around each other, with your remaining fingers free. Pull your thumbs against each other as you exhale and bend slowly to your right. Inhale and return to the upright position. Repeat until you have done seven bends to the right. Rehook your thumbs from the other direction and now bend to the left seven times. Maintain the tension on your thumbs throughout the exercise, then relax with your arms at your sides.

Forward Bends

This exercise provides a good massage of the lymph glands under your arms.

Stand relaxed,with your arms at your sides. Then hook your fingers behind your back, pulling one hand against the other. Stretch your arms out straight. Step forward with your right foot into a wide but comfortable stance. Inhale normally then exhale, bending forward and stretching your arms out straight behind you. As you bend over, lift your arms as high as is comfortable behind you. Maintain the tension between your hands. You may bend your left knee a bit if that seems necessary. Inhale as you return to the upright position, arching back a bit and looking upwards. Repeat for a total of seven bends, then relax.

Now repeat the technique, this time stepping forward with the left foot. Remember that the tension between your hands must be maintained during all seven bends.

Back Bends

Stand relaxed, with your arms at your sides. Bring your hands up and press your palms together in front of your chest. Slowly raise your arms until they are overhead. Inhale and lean backward as far as is comfortable. Maintain the pressure on your palms and hold your breath for a moment. Exhale as you return to the upright position and then continue until you lean slightly forward. Repeat seven times, always maintaining the tension in your arms by pressing your palms tightly together. Relax and let your arms rest at your sides. Be aware that holding the back bend too long may cause you to become lightheaded as you lean forward, so listen to your body in this respect.

Spinal Twist

You should try to do the entire sequence on one inhalation, but if you run out of air, catch a quick sniff. This exercise should not be rushed.

Lie face down on the ground, with your arms at your sides and close to your body. Inhale and slowly raise your torso as you arch your back and look up. At the same time, bring your hands up and place them flat on the ground, just under your shoulders. Continue to inhale as you slowly extend your arms and push your body for more of an arch in your back, as you look up at the ceiling.

Still retaining your breath, slowly twist to one side and look behind you. Return to the front. Twist to the other side and look behind you. Return to the centre.

Exhale, slowly returning to the face down position and returning your arms to your sides. Perform this exercise for ten times, then relax.

❑

24
KNOW YOUR AURA

The idea of a human aura, a relating luminous cloud' surrounding the body is an ancient one. It became so popular in Christian art before the aura was considered an attribute of ordinary everyday morals. For centuries, it has been believed that clairvoyant people could actively see an aura surrounding ordinary visuals, and this aura differed from person to person in Colour and Character, expressing the health, emotional and spiritual attributes of the subject. The visionary Swedenborg wrote in his spiritual diary, "There is a spiritual sphere surrounding everyone as well as a natural and corporeal Aura."

(The Human Aura' by W.J. Miner)

There are 3 major sources of Prana

(*i*) Solar Prana

(*ii*) Air Prana and

(*iii*) Ground Prana

Five elements that compose human body are Air, Heat, Earth, Vacuum and Water and the classifications, as shown above, engulf there of the five elements. To keep our body alive we need life energy (Prana or Ki'). It is known as a 'Pneuma' (in Greek) 'Mana'(in Poynesian) and 'Ruah'(the Hebrew) which means = "the breath of life". In order to rid the patient of his illness, the healer projects 'the health of life (Prana or Ki) to him'. This type of Prana healing is also called 'Miraculous Healing', though there may not seem any miracle in this process.

Solar Prana

It is derived from sunlight and is utilized to promote good health by invigorating the body. One can obtain the solar energy of drinking water exposed in the sun or by sunbathing or even by taking bath in the sun or massaging the body under the sunlight. Since solar energy is extremely potent, the patient must root expose his body too the much to Solar Prana. Certain persons have hypersensitive and tender skin, hence they must be extra cautions while exposing their bodies. Persons, having bilious tendency, ought to be overcautious.

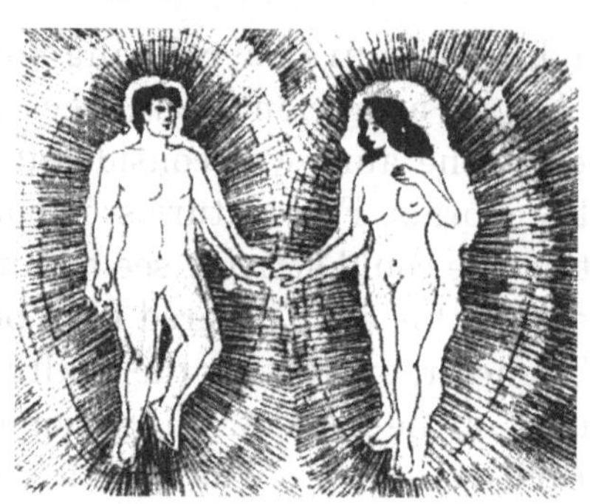

Auras

Air Prana

It is an air vitality globe (Air Prana) which is absorbed by the lungs through breathing as also absorbed directly by the bioplasmic body's energy centres. More volume/quantity of Air Prana can be better absorbed by deep, slow, and rhythmic breathing than by short, rapid and shallow breathing. Certain well trained experts can absorb less energy through the Skin pores.

Ground Prana

It is also called 'ground vitality globe' which is absorbed through soles of the feet (by walking barefoot). It is also absorbed unnoticed, unconsciously or automatically. If one can draw in ground prana to enhance one's vitality, ability to think more correctly, capacity to more work, one should learn to exhausted ground Prana consciouly.

So far, only such factors have been described which help the life energy to activate the diseased organs. First, we have to activate and energise the blocked passages because, as long as such inhibiting factors are not removed, prana energy cannot reach the body, and more particularly to the diseased organs. If the ailment is too chronic and complicated, one has to, naturally, spend more tune to remove the bottleneck. A healer must know which organ is to be energized and what among of life energy is actually needed to affect proper cure. The healer and the patient have to exert patience and perseverance, as there is no room for a complacent approach or half-baked treatment. Further, mental disorders may take morc timc to cure the physical disorders, though direct relationship between mind and physical body cannot be denied.

❑

25
DIVISIONS OF PRANA

These are also called 'Pancha Pranas', that is Prana, Apana, Samana, Udana and Vyana. Now, a brief description of the five sub-Pranas.

1. Prana Vayu: Its field of action is entered around and on heart. It also affects mouth, tongue, throat, nose, eyes and skin. Prana Vayu exerts control over life. Force, heart, mind, salivation, spitting, vomiting, eructations, process of respiration, cough, and also helps to let in food. Vitiation of this vayu causes hiccough and respiratory problems.

2. Udana Vayu: It is seated in the throat, but also exerts its influence upon nose, throat, thorax and umbilicus. It causes and promotes desire/tendency to speak, sing, swallow etc. Its vitiation can cause disorders related to collar bone, larynx (voice box or organ), mouth infections, stammering, dumbness etc.

3. Samana Vayu: It is centred around the navel, but also moves to pubic area and stomach. Its main function lies in promoting digestion, providing requisite aid to quicken the process of food digestion and to segregate juices, faecal matter and urine from the indigestion food-stuff. Its vitiation causes loose motions, colitis, indigestion, wind/gas trouble etc.

4. Apana Vayu: Its field of action is quite wide as it relates to digestive system, including anus, bladder, seminal duct, testicles, pubic region. It helps to facilitate expulsion of faeces, urine, semen, menstrual flow and foetus. When Apana Vayu gets vitiated, obstruction is created in the process of expulsion of the said objects. If Apana Vayu is in order, all other types of Vayu are also in perfect order.

5. Vyana Vayu: This type of Vayu pervades all over the body and controls motions eye-lids, lips, tongue, hands, feet, fingers, genitalia, anus etc. If this Vayu gets vitiated paralysis of single part or whole body takes place. It also must not be forgotten in case of tension, convulsion, retarded mobility etc.

In addition to the above, there are five minor or Upa Pranas:

(*i*) Naga: Responsible for hiccuping and belching

(*ii*) Koorma: It opens the eyes

(*iii*) Krikara: It induces thirst and hunger

(*iv*) Devadatta: It is responsible for Yawning

(*v*) Dhananjaya: It is responsible for the decomposition of the body after death.

❑

26

ELEMENTS OF PRANA AND BREATHING PROCESS

Prana is the sustaining force of human body. As long as prana exists in the body, life persists and, when prana leaves it, death ensues. Right from birth to death, prana is all-pervasive. It is the be-all and end-all of human existence. Prana is nurtured by five elements, viz.

1. Air
2. Water
3. Earth
4. Akash, and
5. Fire

The above mentioned five elements, when in balanced and equilibrium, help the human body to sustain itself but, when this balance is disturbed, a diseased state sets in. Disease is nothing but simply state of a disordered air which is the most predominant factor, as we cannot live or breathe in and breathe out without air, though we can live without the rest of four elements for sometime. Next to Air comes water and then the remaining elements.

Human body is composed of two parts viz.

(*i*) The visible Physical body and

(*ii*) The invisible Energy body (also called 'The Bioplasmic Energy'.)

Visible physical body is that which we touch, see and hear. Bioplasmic body is an invisible luminous energy body that inter penetrates the visible physical body and extends beyond it by 4 to 5 inches and clairvoyants prefer to call the "energy body", "The etheric body" or "etheric double."

Whenever a person is infected by some ailment, his ailing organ/part indicates lack or inadequate energy flow. When the life energy or Ki is replenished, a state of health returns. As long as life energy permeates to each organ and sinew of body, there is hardly any chance of facing any health hazard. The healer transmits life energy to his patient through various means, like psychic healing, therapeutic healing, vitalic healing, magnetic healing, faith healing, charismatic healing. In some cases, some saints and holy men simply rid the patient of his illness by looking deep into his eyes (Which, in fact, is kind of establishment of visual contact between the patient and the healer). In short, a healer projects Prana to the patient.

I would compare Pranic energy to air filling in a tube. If too much air volume is created, the filled in tube can burst and, if too less of air is filled, there are chances the same may get damaged and cracked. There must be reasonable vacuum in a tube so that there is sufficient scope for the air to revolve therein. Let us compare this analogy to human body. When body is overloaded with too much eatables, it gets bloated but, when it is sparsely fed, it creates near starvation position hence, to keep the body in good humour, feed your body only with requisite diet. It is well said, "We are what we eat", that is to say that food choices (or better say 'food preferences') govern our habits and inclinations. If physical body is continuously starved of requisite nutritional diet, it is bound to adversely affect various functions of our body.

Following aspects greatly impact our Pranic efficiency.

1. Process of breathing
2. Five Koshas (or Five sheaths)
3. Chakras
4. Endocrine Glands

5. Nadis-the pathways of Pranic Current
6. Power of Mantras
7. Meridians
8. Disease
9. Food
10. Environmental effects
11. Psychic disorders
12. In-built habits and tendencies
13. Sanskaras
14. Socio-economic and family related problems, including job related problems
15. Personality traits
16. Sex related problems
17. Tendencies like desire, Anger, Avarice, hatred, Attachment, Arrogance, jealousy, contempt, Discrimination etc.

Most of the aspects are interrelated and inter-dependent, but have separate entity also. For instance, when we eat wrong and prohibited food or inhale polluted air, our digestive and respiratory organs' capacity to function adopt a low tone, thereby affecting entire metabolism. Further, tendencies like avarice, anger, hatred, arrogance adversely affect glandular secretions' thereby disturbing our physical chemistry, so on and so forth. Now I will try to explain some of the more conspicuous factors, in the subsequent chapters.

Breathing

Our body functions, generally, in a silent manner without any notice. Breathing is a natural process and we are neither aware nor conscious of this process. Heart-beats, though not noticed generally, indicate our pulse rate. Rapid breathing and strenuous exercise or any activity accelerates pulse rate, with rise in our respiration. When we are tense, ill or agitated or suffer from any mental tension, our heart-beat accelerates and, in order to keep the pulsating of our heart, we have to breathe rapidly so as to keep pace with inspiration and exhalation.

Breathing Process and Organ's Nose

Nose is the chief organ for respiration. It comprises of two Nasal passages, aloe or (two wings which have the capacity to expand and contract). The nostrils have tiny hairs within which sift the harmful substances and allow entry of only pure air into the lungs. Mucous lining in the nose helps to saturate and moisten inhaled air. Septum is a cartilageous bone that divides,two Nasal passages. In Pranayama and yoga the left Nostril is called 'Chandra Nadi' and the right one as 'Surya Nadi'. Two bones, called turbinates, protrude from the side walls of both the nostrils.

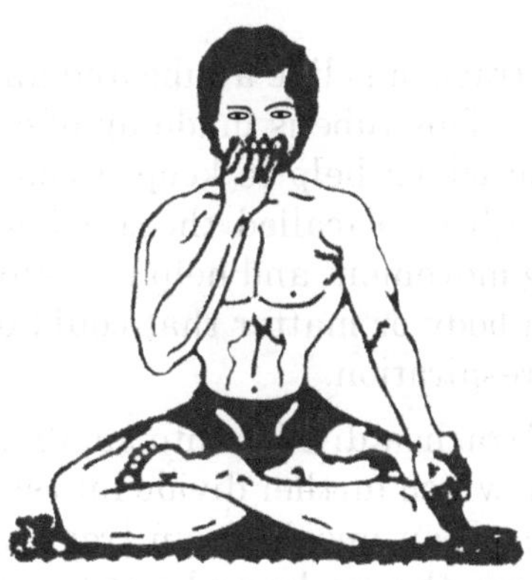

Pranayama

The inhaled air is humidified by the lachrymal fluid which is formed by the glands in the eyes. This fluid continually runs from the eyes to the nose so as to moisten the inhaled air through the nasopharyngeal duct/but, when it comes out of the eyes in the form of tears, when one weeps or has cries, suffers from some sort of infection. The cavaties in the facial bones, called 'Paranasal Sinuses', are connected to the nose. The inhaled air enters these cavities, forming currents that help the dust (inhaled through air) to settle down. Chief functions of the nose lie in purifying, warming and humidifying the inhaled air. This process may be called as 'the air conditioning system' without which lungs would get clogged with dust or else become dry, thereby becoming susceptible to various infections and resultant diseases.

Inhaled Air passes through the pharynx from the nasal cavities. Pharynx lies at the back of the throat where the hard palate terminates. From pharynx the air moves on to the larynx (also called 'Voice box') which commences at the point where food and air passages (respectively known as 'oesophagus' and 'Trachea') conjoin. The larynx contains vocal cords and is made up of cartilage. These vocal cords are emanating source of production of voice. Lower end of the throat gets divided into food passage and air passage, and is flapped by a lid called 'Epiglottis'. When food is eaten and liquid is drunk, the said lid covers the air passage completely so that no food particle could enter therein.

Wind Pipe or trachea is like a tube and air/wind enters into it from the larynx. This tube is made up of cartilaginous rings and muscle tissue which help to keep it constantly open. The trachea is lined with 'Cila' (called 'the tiny hairs' which have an upward sweeping movement and help to remove pollen, dust or any other foreign body or matter that could damage the lungs and also impede respiration.

Lower end of trachea divides into smaller tubes called left and right bronchi, which further divide into smaller bronchioles (like the branches of an upside-down tree). The large branchi retain small and smooth muscles and cartilage that prevent them from closing. As soon as these bronchial tubes become smaller, the cartilage disappears, and only a Celiated muscus lining and fibrous muscular coat are left behind. The bronchioles terminate at small dilated air-tubes (called 'Alveoli') which are lined by capillaries and exchange of oxygen and carbon dioxide takes place between air and blood.

The Lungs

The inner structure of lungs resembles a tree whose main trunk is trachea, bronchi and bronchioles the branches and leaves being the alveoli. There is a lung each on left and right sides of the chest, and lung tissue is pink and coloured (when in an unpolluted state) due to presence of blood capillaries. The left lung has only two lobes/compartments (while the right lung has three lobes) due to the fact that heart occupies room in the left ribcage. Each lung is elastic, spongy and porous, due to the presence of air in its alveoli, as if it floats on water.

The lungs are caged in a ribcage (Thorax) and are separated, from the stomach and other digestive organs, by the diaphragm which lies where the ribs terminate or end. Pleura (double membrane) surrounds the lungs and provides a lubricating surface, between the inner chest cavity and the lungs, during the motions or movements of breathing. Heart sends impure blood to the lungs for oxygenation and expulsion of carbon dioxide. After purifying process, the lungs send back purified and oxygenated blood to the heart to enable it to feed the physical system.

The Rib-cage

This is also called a thoracic cavity, within which heart is contained. The ribcage comprises of bones, muscles and cartilege and helps the air to pump in and pump out. The lungs are passive but have the capacity to inflate and deflate due to the impact of movement of the walls and floor of the thoracic cavity. The thorax is bound by 12 thoracic vertebrae of the spine. The sternum or the breastbone lies in front of the 12 pairs of ribs that encircle the heart and lungs from the vertebral column at the back. The thoracic ribcage protects the vital organs from damage. The spaces between the ribcage contain inter costal muscles that connect them and also impart movement capacity to the ribcage. The ribs are articulated at each end so that they can move outwards and upwards.

The Diaphragm

Diaphragm performs major part of respiration, as ribcage can produce only a limited range of contraction and expansion of lungs. Diaphragm is a dome-shaped organ which has sheet of muscles and tendons attached to the lower ribs, and bulging upwardly into the thoracic cavity. It also forms a dividing partition between thoracic and abdominal cavities. It is an important organ from where oesophagus, vagus nerve and main vein (vena cava) and Artery (Aorta) to and for the lower body, pass through openings in the diaphragm.

On inhalation the diaphragm expands but raises upwardly while, on exhalation, it contracts. During inhalation the abdomen should bloat and expand but contract and squeeze when air is expelled. However, muscular effort is required, in both cases of inhalation and exhalation. Peristaltic Action of the diaphragm massages and stimulates abdominal viscera, helps in digestion, assimilation and excretion.

Breath Volumes (including lung volume)

When we breathe in air, during the course of inhalation, but get impeded breathing, when we inhale about half a litre air, even though full capacity of lungs works to 41/2–5 litres–the former is called 'Tidal Volume and the latter is called 'Vital capacity'. Inhalation and exhalation can be increased/decreased up-and-down the tidal volume. Despite all this, some volume of air always remain in the lungs, even if we feel that entire air volume has been exhaled. This is called 'Residual Volume' which is slightly more than one litre.

When atmospheric air is inhaled, we inhale

- 0.04% Carbon dioxide (which is poison)
- 20% Oxygen (which is body's life force).
- 79% Nitrogen (which doesn't play any role in our respiratory process)

But when air is exhaled following changes are generally noticed, that is

- There is no change in percentage of Nitrogen
- Carbon dioxide increases to around 4.04%. Oxygen is reduced to 16%.

It may be noted that cold air as inhaled and more humid and warm air is exhaled, due to water vapour exhalation from the lungs. During exhalation 1/5th of our body's heat is lost.

Respiration

The term 'Respiration' implies both the processes of inhalation and exhalation. Breathing is a natural phenomenon and pace of breathing varies from one person to another. Normally an adult breathes 15 breaths per minute which number can increase or decrease in view of one's physical, emotional and mental states as also due to environmental influences. Nervous and chemical controls are the two factors that control and regulate air respiratory mechanism.

Breathing is a natural, silent and uninterrupted process. When breathing process is in order, everything else is in perfect order but, when breathing process is disturbed, nothing else can be in order, as a body without breath is a dead entity. If, we, have to survive, we have to breathe so that oxygen is supplied to the body to let it function normally. The marvel of breathing lies in continuous and unemployed breathing, as we continue to breathe, even if we are asleep or awake. When we are asleep, the subconscious mind supervenes but, during activity or awakened state conscious mind takes control of our body. This fact will be laid open and discussed, in greater details, when dealing with 'Pranayama'.

Nose and its Utility

Imagine what would be the condition of any person when both the nostrils get blocked, due to accumulation of thick, tenacious and sticky mucocus, and one is obliged to breathe through mouth. When one has to breathe through mouth, tongue and throat membranes get dried up. Moreover, mouth breathing is only an emergent device and can never replace nasal breathing. Further, during mouth breathing all the foreign matters gain entry into our body.

Nose is the only organ that imparts us sense of smell and also helps to build up taste and liking for food. Nose has a direct connection with our brain, and its nostrils are the doorways that affect our entire mental and physical systems. Respiration gets impeded, if nostrils are blocked or choked. In order to facilitate breathing, without any hassles, try to keep your nasal passages clear by Pranayama, deep breathing, 'Neti Kriya', or steam inhalation. If nasal passages get frequently blocked yard respiration becomes a problem, seek help of a yoga expert.

If you have a blocked nose, you are most likely to develop catarrhal headache which may even percolate to eyes, temples, neck, check bones, sinuses. If there are hard crusts in the nose do not remove them forcibly, as you are likely to cause nasal bleeding and resultant wounds. Constant discharge or flow or obstruction may even damage septum and cartilages. Clear your nasal passages with saline water (cold or lukewarm). For free respiration, nasal passages must be free from all types of obstructions, including polypi, crusts, thick and tenacious mucous which is difficult to detach.

The Respiratory System

"The Respiratory System enables oxygen from the air to be taken into the bloodstream to provide the energy to the body to meets its needs to function. As we breathe in, air is filtered by the nose, then travels via the windpipe (trachea) and bronchial tubes to the lungs, into millions of tiny sacs. Oxygen passes through the thin sac walls into the blood, in exchange for carbon dioxide, a waste product, which is breathed out. Mucous may collect in little–used parts of the lungs, encouraging bacteria to grow. In urban areas the air is often laden with chemicals from industry and traffic, placing a strain on the respiratory mucous membranes' defences.

Treatment aims to reduce the intake of pollutants and allergens, and lessen their effects on the lungs. Building up the immune system helps the body resist attack by micro-organisms inhaled through the nose and mouth.

Infections of the respiratory tract are often triggered by viruses. Irritation of the mucous membranes may constrict the airways, making breathing difficult. Decongestants, antihistamines and broncho-dilators may be prescribed. Any secondary bacterial infections (those which occur after viral infections) are treated using antibiotics.

Air inhaled via the nose or mouth enters the windpipe (trachea) in the throat. The trachea divides into two tubes (bronchi) which enter the lungs–spongy, elastic air-filled organs to either side of the heart. Within each lung, the bronchi branch into smaller aid smaller tubes. The very smallest tubes (bronchioles) carry air into tiny sacs (alveoli) which are surrounded by microscopically fine blood vessels (capillaries), whose walls are so thin that oxygen from the air easily diffuses through them and into the red blood corpuscles, where it is carried in haemoglobin to body tissues. The respiratory tract is lined with mucous membranes.

The Theory of Relaxation and Breathing

With each breath, oxygen is absorbed into the blood, enabling production of the energy that fuels every body function. Under stress, breathing tends to be rapid, using the top half of the lungs. This causes a drop in blood levels of carbon dioxide, whiter is needed to maintain blood acidity. This can lead to tiredness and anxiety and create tension in the upper back, shoulders and neck. Abdominal breathing, which allows the lungs to expand full is a more efficient and calm way to breathe, and has the potential to benefit both physical and mental health.

Abdominal Breathing

Abdominal, or diaphragmatic, breathing uses the diaphragm the sheet of muscle that forms the floor of the chest cavity and the ceiling of the abdomen. On breathing in, the diaphragm contracts and moves downward rather like the piston of a bicycle pump. At the same time, the abdomen rises and the chest expands slightly as air is drawn in. On breathing out, the diaphragm relaxes and rises, making the space inside the chest cavity smaller and expelling air from the lungs.

How Oxygen Reaches the Bloodstream

As air is drawn into the lungs, alveoli (air sacs) transfer oxygen into the bloodstream and remove carbon dioxide from it.

Physiological Effects of Stress and Relaxation

Stressful situations trigger the body's fight-or-flight response to stress. If stress persists, mental and physical health are undermined, partly because the stress hormones, adrenaline and cortisol, interfere with functioning of the circulatory and immune systems. Relaxation combats many of these effects.

Response to Stress

Adrenaline is released into bloodstream; heart-.rate and blood pressure increase.

Liver releases energy, stored as glycogen; blood-sugar and cholesterol levels increase.

Faster breathing; increased metabolic rate.

Muscular tension; increased production of lactic acid.

Gastric acid increases or decreases; digestive enzymes and inhibited peristals is Perspiration increases.

Increased levels of cortisol; immune system inhibited.

Emotional tension; as attention is focused on emergency reaction.

Long-Term Effects of Stress

High blood pressure; anxiety; insomnia; irritability

High cholesterol levels.

Breathlessness; hyperventilation; palpitations.

Muscular aches and pains, including headaches and backpain.

Nausea; indigestion; constipation; ulcers; food intolerances.

Skin rashes; eczema.

Raised cortisol levels increase the risk of problems in the immune system.

Emotional outbursts; depression.

Responses to Relaxation.

Decreased adrenaline levels; lower blood pressure; less stress on cardiovascular system, Decreased blood sugar and cholesterol levels, Slower breathing improved lung function and metabolic rate.

Relaxed musclesless lactic acid in muscles.

Improved digestive process.

Improved physiological stability.

Increased activity of immune system; less susceptibility to illness.

Emotional calm; increased alertness and energy.

❑

27
BREATHING SCIENCE

Prana means the vital force or life energy and yama means to control. Hence, pranayama means to control the vital energy by control of breath or the breathing process. But the question arises what is prana? What is the need of regulation of prana and what are its benefits?

The breathing process goes on in the body, since birth till death. The process of inhaling air and exhaling is called breathing. Prana is that inner energy, that is present in all animate and inanimate matter. Hence, the air, we breathe, is different from the prana. Air, we take in, has a gross form, while prana has a subtle form.

The two bases of this creation are–akaga (ether) and prana (vital life force). Both are omnipresent. The vibrance of the vital life force in the ether led to creation. Prana or vital life force is, thus, said to be before the creation of the mind.

The scriptures have elucidated the practice of pranayama for controlling the mind. Prana is the omnipresent vital life force that energises and spurs the mind. We take in prana through the breath. Taking a deep breath fills the three parts of lungs with pranic energy. These three parts are the upper part upto the neck, the parts on both sides of the heart and lower parts. Besides this, the pranic energy even starts to flow to the navel region, when we take deep breath. If we do not inhale-exhale, properly, or if we do not perform pranayama, these parts remain deprived of the vital energy. Through the blood, pranic energy is transferred to all parts of the body. Following are some verses from the ancient texts, elucidate the importance of pranic energy.

The Rigveda States

All living beings that live from the mountains to the ocean, breathe air in two ways only–inhale and exhalle. If these are mastered, then all the six sense-organs will work, harmoniously.

After mastering postures, by retention of inhalation and exhalation, one should practice the science of breathing called pranayama.

In fact, all ancient Indian texts, like the Vedas and the Smrtis, elucidate the importance of pranayama.

There are seven centres in the human body, through which the pranic energy is transferred into the various parts of the body. These centres are called chakras, i.e., psychic centres. If even one chakra is in a state of imbalance, the body is stricken by some ailment or the other. Pranayama is important for bringing up and maintaining this balance. In spiritual terms, it is the path to total emanciation.

Although in this physical body, the pranic energy is in one form, but, according to the different activities in the body, the prana divides itself into five main divisions. These are called pailca pranas. There are further five sub-divisions of prana, called the pailca upapranas.

The five divisions are prana, apana, samana, udana and vyana, while the sub-divisions are naga, Kurma, Krkala, devadatta, dhananjaya.

The age, to which a human being can be expected to live, can be determined by the pranic energy, derived by him through breathing. Those who breathe shallow and quick live a shorter life span in comparison to those who breathe, deep and slow. The ancient is his studied the different animals and came to this conclusion. As snakes, elephants and tortoises have a slow rate of breathing, they have a longer life span. While animals like dogs, rabbits and birds which have a fast breathing rate are short-lived. Hence, through pranayama, one cannot just have physical and spiritual benefits, rather one could enhance one's life span. The following table would show how the rate of breathing has a direct effect on one's life span.

1. Tortoise 4-5 times per minute life span–200 years
2. Snake 7-8 times per minute life span–150 years
3. Man 15-16 times a minute life span–100 years
4. Horse 20-22 times a minute life span–40 years
5. Dog 28-30 times a minute life span–14 years

The text, Svara Yoga, explains what the effect would be when the exhaled air is thrown out at a certain distance. Normally, in rechaka or exhalation, the breath, coming out, can be felt at a distance of twelve fingers from the nostrils. While puraka or inhalation can be felt ten fingers away. If the recka is felt 11 fingers away, then, the pranic energy gets stabilized; 10 fingers, one gets peace and happiness; 9 fingers ,one becomes a poet; 8 fingers, one becomes eloquent; 7 fingers breadths, one becomes foresighted; 6 fingers breadths, one becomes capable of flying in the sky; 5 fingers, one can travel at the speed of thought; 4 fingers, one gains the eight siddhis or spiritual powers (supra) normal powers; 3 fingers, one comes to possess the nine nidhis, i.e., treasures or the keys to worldly prosperity; 2 fingers, one becomes capable of assuming several physical forms at the same time; 1 finger, one can become invisible; 1/ 10th of 1 finger, one conquers death.

In different activities, rechka has the following force:

normal state	–	upto 6 fingers
emotional state	–	upto 12 fingers
singing	–	upto 16 fingers
eating	–	upto 20 fingers
walking	–	upto 24 fingers
sleeping	–	upto 30 fingers
sexual activity and exercising	–	36 fingers

All this explanation has been given to make one understand the importance of pranayama. One can control the speed and depth of the breathing for physical and spiritual gains.

It is through the prana, i.e., the vital life force, that one can form a link between the body and the soul. Hence, prana is the link between the gross and the subtle world. A body, without

Prana, is usually declared dead and one could say that the *Soul* has left for the heaven.

First of all, pranayama keeps the body healthy and, secondly, it keeps the mind, still and concentrated. If the pranic energy keeps flowing, continuously and unhindered, through the susumna channel related to kundalini, then, the path to spiritual progress opens up for the person. Pranayama also increases the sexual power, Through celibacy, pure-balanced diet and pranyama, one could enhance one's mental powers, as well. Through pranayama, even though restricted by the medium of this small physical form, being in this physical body, one can possess all the divine powers of the universe, as it is, and also, in their true form.

Pranayama affects the entire body system and tones the blood circulation, glandular system, nervous system, pranic energy channel network, the store of pranic energy in the body and the subtle body.

❑

28
GUIDELINES FOR PRANAYAMA

- One should practise pranayama in an airy, open, well-ventilated place. One should not practise it in a room filled with dust, smoke, dampness, bad odour and rubbish. One should, also not try in very fast blowing wind.
- One should try on an empty stomach or four hours after meals or half an hour before meals.
- One should wear clothes according to the season but they should not be very tight.
- It is best to practise early in the morning. In winters, one could also try at noon or in the evening.
- Practise pranayama after Yoga postures and before meditation.
- During pranayama, keep the body relaxed and loose.
- Sit on a folded blanket, covered with a cotton cloth, for pranayama. Sit in any meditative pose.
- One can practise more during winters than summers.
- Do not practise bhastrika and suryabhedi, during summers. In winters, refrain from practising sitali, sitkari and chandrabhedi pranayama.
- Those suffering from asthma, high blood pressure, hypertension and heart problems should not practise kumbhaka without the proper guidance of an expert.
- Do not put extra force on the body, during pranayama. Hold the breath, only as long as it is comfortable. Otherwise, it might create an adverse effect on the lungs.

- Those practising pranayama, should avoid smoking, tobacco, meat and alcohol.
- Those with wind humour predominant should not practise and those with bile humour dominant should not practise suryabhedi and those with phlegm predominant should not practise chandrabhedi pranayama.
- Suryabhedi cures imbalance of wind, humour, ujjayr cures phlegm, imbalance, Sitali and Sitkari cure bile imbalance while Mastrika cures the imbalance of all the three.
- One should practise asanas after having a bath. Otherwise, one should bathe half an hour after the practice.
- If one starts sweating, instead of wiping it off with a towel, one should massage with the hands and dry it off or let it dry off, naturally.
- If one is suffering from cold or the nostrils are blocked, then, one should not practise pranayama.
- One should not break the practice, again and again. Otherwise, the benefits cannot be attained, fully, and will not last long.

For the practice of pranayama, one should understand the breathing process, properly. Breathing can be of two types– abdominal breathing and chest breathing.

Udara Svasana (Abdominal Breathing)

Lie down on the floor on your back like the corpse-pose and place one hand's palm on the navel. Inhale deeply in a way that the abdomen bellows like a balloon and rises. The more the navel region rises the diaphragm goes down. Diaphragm is the tissue wall that separates the lungs from the abdomen.

Next, exhale slowly. For this, contract the abdomen and allow the hand on the navel to go downwards, rather push it towards the spine. As the abdominal region contracts, the chest expands.

Keep the chest and shoulders still during the practice. Repeat 10 to 15 times.

Urah Svasana (Chest Breathing)

Sit with crossed legs or lie down. Expanding the chest, breathe in deeply. If necessary, place the hands on the waist with the thumbs positioned on the back, while the rest of the fingers on your stomach and, then, with the rest of the fingers, press the stomach in.

Exhale i.e. perform rechaka, allowing the chest to sink in. Inhale i.e. perform puraka, allowing only the chest to expand. In this practice, do not expand or contract the stomach. Repeat 5 to 10 times.

Both the above practices are very good for the health of any person. Generally, as one is not able to breathe, deeply, in this manner in the normal course. These preparatory practices of pranayama are necessary for good health and longevity too.

Purna Svasana or Yogic Svasana

(Yogic Breathing)

Sitting in any comfortable posture raise the hands above the head and place the arms on the back from above the shoulders. Push back the elbows by your head. Thus, the ribs will be stretched and the chest will expand to the maximum. Expanding both the chest and the abdomen, fill the lungs with air, performing paraka. After this, relaxing the abdomen and the chest, perform recaka or exhale. In the end, by pressing the abdomen and contracting the chest, expel all the air present in the lungs. The entire practice should be rhythmic and not in jerks.

Pranayama is described in two parts here, (a) Preparatory practices of pranayama, (b) Pranayama.

❑

29

PRANAYAMA: METHOD AND BENEFITS

By the term Pranayama is meant regulation of Prana and its distribution to various parts of the body. Pranayama is performed by

(*i*) Manipulation of respiration beyond its normal limit. (H) Stretching it.

(*iii*) Flowing it down so as to experience the full range of respiration of gross and subtle levels.

Pranayama is Performed by Following Methods

- By inhaling the breath in quick succession and then exhaling.
- By inhaling Prana (air or life energy) by one nostril and exhalation through the other.
- By inhalation of Prana through both the nostrils, retain the same as per one's capacity and then releasing the same gradually, until the stomach is fully emptied.
- While inhaling the stomach should inflate and lungs contract or squeeze.
- While exhaling stomach should get drown in or squeezed and lungs expanded.
- Quick respiration, resembling bellow of a black snuth.
- By throwing out prana forcefully and then inhaling the same.
- By sudden stoppage or suspension of breath and then retaining the residual part thereof within the body as per one's capacity.

During meditation normal breathing should be maintained and mind should be concentrated upon breathing and wayward thoughts should be controlled. To perform Pranayama an aspirant can sit in any convenient asana (sitting posture) like Padmasana, Swastikasana, Siddhasana or simply squat on the floor, bed or even sit in a chair or sofa, as an inconvenient posture will not allow your mind to concentrate.

Rhythmic Respiration (Breathing)

In natural breathing no discomfort is felt, and natural/normal breathing is another nomenclation of rhythmic breathing which differs in case of every person.

Variations in Breathing Process

(*i*) Irregular breathing indicates tension.

(*ii*) Shallow and rapid breathing is indicative of anxiety.

(*iii*) Forceful and short breathing means state of anger.

(*iv*) Relaxed state of body and mind indicates a rhythmic, slow and smooth respiration.

(*v*) Gaspeng and arrhythmic breathing indicates a state of grief.

(*vi*) When there is irregular breathing, it indicates disturbed mental states and neurosis.

(*vii*) Breathing can even be incomplete and uneven in certain types of neurosis.

(*viii*) Slow rhythmic breathing is believed to impact and create feelings of relaxation, reduced muscle tension and alpha brain waves.

To begin with, try to tune into the rhythms of breath and align the same with the outside world. This, invariably, includes, heart beat, brain rhythms, mental emotional, emotive (emotional) and mental rhythms, wakefulness and sleep etc. but there are always variations in intensity and frequency. All such rhythms occur in relation to changes in weather conditions, mental states, seasons, months, years, and planetary influences. Generally, we are not aware of presence of rhythmic force within our body and mind but Pranayama leads and helps us to realise such rhythmic forces. Constant and regular practice of pranayama can help us to know the changes occurring within the body and also know as to where we are lacking and where improvement is required. A trained mind can help to control such mechanisms so that areas of consciousness and control, (which are generally not within our control) can be unravelled.

Kriyas and Pranayama

Following terms are often used in relation to inhalation, retention and expulsion/release/exhalation of breath (Prana).

1. **Poorak Kriya:** Process of inhalation.
2. **Kumbrak Kriya:** To retain or control.
3. **Rechak Kriya:** Exhalation of breath.

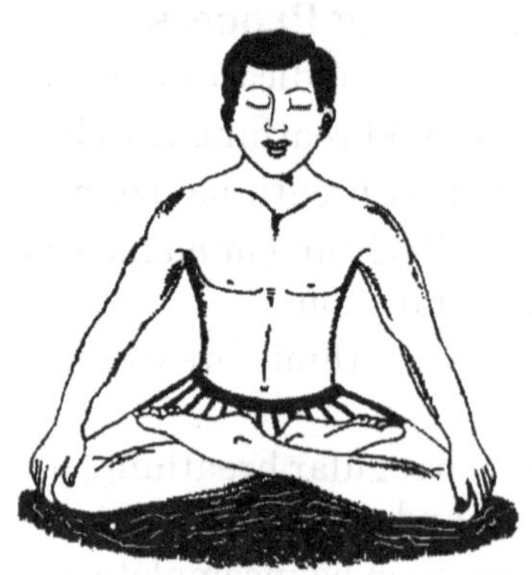

Meditation

If prana/vayu is inhaled but not exhaled, suffocation, laboured breathing, choking may be felt. Hence any breath that is inhaled has to be exhaled so as to avoid discomforts. Moreover, after quick succession of inhalation and exhalation, gap is necessary so as to relax the overworked organs. One has to keep balance between inhaled and exhaled air or Prana, as deficient inspiration will not suffice to nurture the body as a whole and excessive inspiration will overtax our system.

Yogic postures are not simply physical exercises, they are much more than that-they ensure and fortify mental tendencies, faculties, provide succour to your agitated mind and nerves and strengthen your body. Due to space crunch, it is not possible to give a detailed account of all faces of yoga which is science in itself. These are neither physical exercises nor body building devices, nor do with so called modern health clubs, health points, gyms, slimming and weight-loss clinics nor are they source of delight for the elite or pseudo rich classes, they are meant to purify body and mind, provide alacrity, suppleness, agility, peace and tranquillity to mind, to divert the body from diseased states and also to impart immunity from diseases and infections, to arouse body's defence mechanisms.

Pranayama

Pranayama literally means pause during respiration but actually it means control over inhalation and exhalation process. It is the only method by which you can quite easily tone up your entire body, regulate circulation of blood, normalise respiration, increase your heart-beats as also slow down cardiac rhythm by sheer control, let blood reach even the minutest blood vessels and, above all, it requires minimal effort. Pranayama also brings under control your wayward thoughts, keeps you away from worry and tension, imparts sobriety and tranquility to your agitated temperament.

The readers should go through this chapter carefully and, after studying the same, they would find that most of their mental and physical problems have been addressed to and solved. So, without categorising or nomenclating a particular disease and its causative symptom(s) an easy, but effective way, has been suggested. Pranayama has been dealt with under the following 8 classifications, viz.

1. Suryabhedi
2. Ujjayi,
3. Sitkari,
4. Shitali,
5. Bhastrika,
6. Bharamari,
7. Moorchha, and
8. Plavini.

Three terms would be quite frequently used here. Inhalation (Rechaka), Suspension or withholding (Kumbhak) and Release (Poorak) of breath.

❑

30
HEALING THROUGH PRANAYAMA

The breath which enters our body from without (outside) is called 'Shwas' or inhalation of air, and that which goes out from our body is called exhalation or 'Prashawas'. Breath is the life force or vital force or, still better, the sustaining force of our body. Proper balance between inhalation, retention and exhalation forms the very basis of our life (Jeevan). Death is nothing other than existence of this process. It is also subtly called 'Prana'. Pranayama is divided into three stages.

(1) **Poorak:** The terms implies inhalation of air (breath) or inspiration.

(2) **Kumbhak:** It means withholding of breath.

(3) **Rechak:** The term is indicative of exhalation of breath.

Procedure of Pranayama

It is, in fact, a practice for complete respiration. Sit in Padmasana or Sukhasana (lotus pose). Keep your spinal chord erect. Inhale fresh air though the nose, filling your abdomen with the air. When the abdomen is full (by inhalation of air) and bloates, retain the breath as long as you can, without suffocating choking, tiring or straining yourself. Now slowly exhale the air. While inhaling the lungs would contract and the abdomen bloat but when air is exhaled, the abdomen will squeeze and lungs expand. Entire process is called respiratory process. Ratio between all the three stages (Poorak, Kumbhak and Rechak) should preferably be 1:2:1 but there are no hard and fast rules or guidelines. Pranayama can be done even while you are walking, moving on foot or in a vehicle, sitting in a chair (preferably) easy chair, lying down or standing. The only common factor of utmost importance being that the air inhaled must be fresh and pure. If Pranayama done is a choked, smoky, dusty, polluted and toxic environs, it will cause harm, and there is no wonder you may expose your body to various serious disorders.

How to Do Pranayama

Our nose has two nostrils, the left one is called 'Chandra Nari' and the right one is called 'Surya Nari'. One denotes cool and the other heat, one is active at night while the other is active during the day. When we inhale the breath is cold but, when exhale, it is hot. There are certain ascetics who can easily forecast death time of a person from the determination of breathing process, time and speed of breathing as, after all, it is the breath which is the vital force of our moods, climatic changes, etc. Lunar and solar phases and eclipses affect changes in nature, world events, lives of all persons, etc. First of all breath through one nostril only, closing the other with the index finger of your hand. Now retain the breath as long and as conveniently you can. There after, slowly breath out the finger. Before you exhale, the nostril, through which you had breathed should be closed. After a reasonable pause, now following the same process from the other nostril. Inhalation and breathing processes should be slow and uniform.

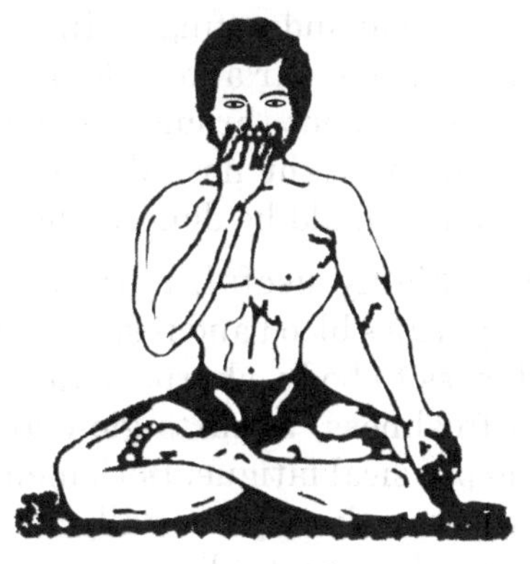

Pranayama

Benefits of Pranayama

As already discussed, pranayama aims at fortifying, sustaining and nurturing vital force of the body. It is connected more with our mental faculties than physical. It corrects various, if not all, physical disorders, by training the mind in such a way that body is rendered strong enough to take the oddities and abnormalities of life and other upsets in normal way, and upheavals and disturbances fail to have any impact on body. It removes defects and abnormalities of eyes, senses of hearing, smell, touch, speech, and purifies blood, normalises breathing process, tones up digestive organs, improves appetite, activates functioning of secretary glands, retards old age, takes away all evil feelings, recharges mental faculties. Above all, it provides peace (mental), sense of satisfaction, happiness and bliss. This is an asana to improve your life span. Recharge your emotions and other activities, by doing it regularly.

Kinds of Pranayama

There are eight kinds of Pranayama viz. (1) Surya-Bhedan, (2) Ujjayi, (3) Sitkari, (4) Shitali, (5) Bhastrika, (6) Bhramari, (7) Moorchha and (8) Plavini. Hereunder, brief description and benefits of each Kriya are described.

Surya-Bhedan

It pertains to perform pranayama through the Surya-Nari (Right Nostril). Sit in Padma, Sidha or Swastikasana. Inhale fresh air through the right nostril, closing the left nostril (Chandra Nari) with your index finger. Inhaled breath should be suspended or retained as far and as long as possible. Before suffocation sets in, breath out through the left nostril, keeping your index finger on the right nostril. The trinity of Poorak, Kumbhak and Rechak should be done without any discomfort.

Benefits: It is highly useful, particularly in winter. It improves appetite, purifies blood and respiratory system, imparts agility and suppleness to body, sharpens and purifies memory, gives a feeling of freshness, imparts glow and lustre to body, dispels mental and physical fatigue. Both men and women of all ages are advised to do this Pranayama daily but more particularly in winter to let the body get vital heat.

Ujjayi

Sit in Padma, Sidha or Swastikasana (whichever suits you as the most comfortable and easy). Expel forcibly the air from the body. While expelling breath, there must be the sound which is heard during sleep, as if you are expelling air during sleep. Thereafter, inhale fresh air to the full capacity of your lungs, expanding your chest as far as you can. In this pranayama, breath is not to be retained. When you feel lungs are fully filled with air release/breath out the air slowly, making sure that during the course of expelling air, there is natural own of exhalation process.

Benefits: The process can be done while walking, writing, sitting, getting up. It modifies heat (excessive) in the body, improves secretion of digestive juices, increases appetite, removes constipation, cough and other respiratory disorders. Also provides lustre to the body. It should be performed daily by people of both sexes, irrespective of age.

Sitkari

Be seated in Swastika, Padma or Sidha asana. Let your tongue stay in-between both the rows of teeth. Now slightly clinch your teeth but very gently and softly, so that tongue is not unduly put under pressure of the teeth, both rows should simply touch the tongue so that it does not slip or retrace. Keep your lips open. Now take a deep breath through the mouth, creating a 'hissing' sound (The soul as created by a snake). Retain the breath as far as feasible. Thereafter exhale through the nose very slowly.

Benefits: This exercise is highly beneficial during hot days as it not only dispels ill effects of heat but imparts cooling effect to the body. It modifies excessive bile, improves appetite, dispels lethargy and renders body beautiful. Does not let teeth decay and also promotes general health and texture of teeth. It also induces natural and own sleep. Ladies can also perform this asana.

Shitali

Lengthwise twist the tongue in the form of a crow's beak (or resembling a crow's beak) and slightly protrude the tongue out of lips. Now breathe in through the tongue. Retain the breath by closing your mouth. Do not allow breath to escape out. Before a suffocating tendency surfaces, exhale fully the breath and relax.

Benefits: It is almost a panacea for all types of fever. Also cures all the stomach disorders. All men and women can do it.

Bhastrika

Be seated in a comfortable position (whether in Sidha or Padma asana). Now inhale through both the nostrils in the same way as air in the willow of a black-smith is filled in and eased out. Breathing in and breathing out process, must create an identical sound as comes from the willow. While drawing in breath, your belly should bloat but, while blowing out, your belly should squeeze. Whenever you feel suffocated, exhale through the right nostril. Now repeat the process through the left nostril other process remaining unchanged. Entire process should be done in alteration.

Benefits: Yogis perform this process to awaken Kundalini. It activates digestive juices, thereby arousing natural appetite, removes disorders of the three humours (wind, bile and phlegm), cures and rectifies all throat diseases, does away with cough and asthma, imparts strength and energy to heart and regulated functioning thereof, modifies and normalises pulmonary, respiratory processes improves circulation of blood by activating blood vessels.

Bhramari

Sit in Sidha, Padma or Swastik asana, keeping your spine erect. Inhale through the left nostril, while inhalation create sound like that of a big black bee (Bhramara). Retain breath as long and as you conveniently can. Thereafter slowly exhale through the right nostril.

Benefits: It clears obstruction in the nose, removes heavy feeling in the head, facilitates breathing through nose, pacifies wayward mental attitudes, keeps mind under happiness and transquillity. It will calm down and pacify mental agitation, if performed daily in the evening.

Moorchha

This should be performed while sitting in a Sidhasana as it is a bit difficult posture. Before deciding to practically perform this asana, it is imperative that full guidance is sought from a yoga expert, otherwise it can do more harm than good. Only those, whether ladies or gents, who are desirous to perform it, should have a strong will to follow the rigid norms and follow the complexities before harping on the process. Relevant process is detailed hereunder.

First of all, be seated in Siddhasana. Take a deep breath through both the nostrils. Now retain in the breath, your chin rested on the hollow position of throat (as is done in a Jalandhar Bhandha). Two fingers close to your thumbs (index and middle fingers) of both hands should be delicately placed and rested on your both eyes (over the upper lids). Keep both eyes closed (right eye, with right hand fingers and left eye with left hand fingers). Place the four fingers of both hands on either side of each nose, thus closing both the nostrils. Now the small fingers should be placed just below the lower left, lifting the lower lip so that the same is raised so much that it joins the upper lip (that is when mouth is closed with the help of two little fingers). Now apply the process of 'Mool Bandh' (by stretching your anus and rectum upwards) and 'Udyan Bandha'. Before you start suffocating, release and remove the fingers and exhale through both the nostrils.

Benefits: It pacifies wayward mind, helps in concentrating mind, removes diseases pertaining to blood, skin and respiration. It preserves semen, all stomach and digestive problems disappear. There is no night discharge. Digestion improves, body is infused with extra energy. 'Mool Bandha' helps to awaken the kundalini. It is not recommended for ladies.

Plavini

Sit in Padmasana and inhale (fresh) air so that stomach is filled to its filling capacity. Bloat your abdomen as much as you can. Now exhale the breath. This process be repeated 4-5 times. Before you breath in again, make sure that your abdomen contracts completely after you have exhaled.

Benefits: Renders the entire body supple and light, cleans the bowels in such a way that digestion stands improved, disorders like pile, gas accumulation, extra fat from and around abdomen is shed. It improves figure of a person in general. It is claimed that any person who becomes an adopt in this process may float over water like a lotus, swim or even walk on the water, even if turbulent.

Breathing Exercises

Breathing with rhythm–Sit cross-legged on the ground or on a chair or stand with folded hand as in prayer. Keep mouth closed and breathe in through the nostrils counting one to four. Hold breath till you count from one to eight. Start to breathe out. While breathing out count once again from one to four, hold breath till you count from five to eight before you start inhaling. Repeat this a few more times. Increase the number of counts while breathing in and out and in between, gradually from day to day, to draw in more oxygen and expel more carbon-di-oxide.

Cleansing Pranayama

Sit cross-legged on the ground or on a chair with the spine erect and muscles relaxed. Cover the right nostril with the thumb and inhale through the left nostril. Cover the left nostrils too with the index finger and hold breath for one to two counts. Release the thumb and exhale through the right nostril. Repeat this with the left nostril. Cover the left nostril with the index finger and inhale rough the right. Close both the nostrils and hold for one or two counts and then exhale through the left nostril releasing the index finger. With regular practice the number of counts while holding the breath should increase.

This exercise corrects the disorders of the nasal cavity and lungs. The good supply of oxygen help purify the lungs.

Note: Those who suffer from blood pressure must not practice to hold the breath. They can simply inhale and exhale.

One other Exercise: Sit in a comfortable position with crossed legs. Keep the body relaxed and erect. Keep the mouth closed. Inhale fast as much air as possible and exhale quickly with force. Do not hold the breath but breathe in and out in quick succession. Relax a while, breathing normally and again start breathing in and out in quick succession. Do this five to six times in the beginning and slowly increase after a few days practice.

This exercise is recommended in all digestive and respiratory disorders. It corrects defective circulation.

❑

31
POINTS BEFORE STARTING YOGIC EXERCISES

Of all the complementary or alternate therapies yoga is the most cost effective, holistic, curative, hassle-free and easy-to-perform. It not only purifies body, mind and intellect but, apart from that, it strives to improve digestive, respiratory, cardiac and circulatory, endocrine glands' functioning, mobility and sleeplessness of joints and muscles, renders body slim and trim by helping it to shed extra fat from the body, activates sebaceous glands to keep the skin glazed and sparkling, improves health of ovaries, controls senses. I have mentioned only some of the benefits.

Yogasanas are not aerobic or physical exercises, or work-up for sportsmen and athletes, but much more than that. There is hardly any mental and physical disorder (Dosha or Roga) which it cannot cure, of course it has to be coupled with Pranayama Kriyas to derive optimum and near complete mileage. Readers are advised to go through the following points carefully so that no room is left for confusion.

Yoga and Food

Yoga lays great stress on pure non-irritant, spice free, anti-toxicant, and fresh seasonal vegetable and fruits. Hence, pure vegetarian diet is an integral part of this unique system. Try to avoid fried, saucy, spicy, fat-enriched diet which interferes not only with normal functioning of body organs but also disturbs our mental faculties, thinking, secretions from endocrine glands–in a way all these factors are health hazards. It has been rightly said that 'we are what we eat' which clearly implies that our food patterns and dietary habits not only govern our body but also our thinking process. When our body is ailing, mind is bound to get disturbed, as healthy mind stays only in a healthy body and, in order to keep our body in a healthy state, our diet must be 'Sattvik'. For instance, if a person consumes much of spicy and fat-enriched food, alcohol, tobacco, drugs, his digestive system is bound to get disturbed, resulting in many digestion related disorders.

Yoga and Mind

Mind is the driving force of all our actions. If mind is vitiated, polluted and disturbed, our endocrine glands won't function normally–there will be lessor or more secretion from such glands which will adversely affect our body chemistry. Yoga strives to pacify agitated mental process, thereby imparting it peace, tranquillity and satiation. Yogic postures assist the brain to put in better performance, by nurturing its nerves with the requisite blood supply to sustain and fortify its various activities. Mind is an abstract form of brain and whatever thoughts arise therein are expressed by emotions, sensations, physical actions/reactions.

Yoga and Pranayama

Pranayama means suspension or withholding of breath or regulation of breath through inhalation. Suspension (withholding) and exhalation, and these three phases are part and parcel of all the yogic postures (Asanas). There is life as long as we breath and death ensues only when last breath comes out of our body. If one is able to retain breath, the time saved through retention, adds to longevity of life. Prana is nothing other than breath, hence in order to add to years, one must learn how to preserve expense of breath.

Yogasanas are designed in such a way that entire body's functions get normalised, breathing process regulated, quality of life improved and general well-being of body, mind and intellect ensured. A person who practises yogasanas and Pranayama with punctual regularity can be rest assured to lead a healthy, physical and mental life.

All asanas cannot and must not be performed by all, due to variable disorders and an individual's physical capacity, but Pranayama can be practised by all persons, irrespective of age, sex and physical condition.

Multiple Benefits of Yogasanas

Asanas have multiple benefits, as detailed hereunder:

(1) With certain safeguards and cautions, all men, women and children can perform asanas, depending upon an individual's age, health status or particular diseases from which a person is suffering.

(2) They are easy, cost-effective, preventive, corrective and curative of almost all the disorders, mental or physical or both, and no extra material is required to perform them.

(3) They help in muscle and tissue build-up and repair thereof, apart from calming down agitated nerves, dispelling fatigue, making up for the lost energy. They help to keep body and mind in good humours.

(4) They energise the endocrine glands so that the body receives requisite sections which are vital and necessary for proper functioning of the body.

(5) Digestive system is rejuvenated, appetite improved, digestion related diseases are cured.

(6) It is the best method to keep and sustain flexibility of the spine and remove curvature, if any. In addition, it also rectifies posture-related diseases like back pain, shoulder pain, cervical spondylosis, lumbar spondylosis, joint pains, stiffness of joints etc.

(7) Asanas help to reduce weight, by naturally shedding extra flesh from the body.

(8) The sharpen intellect, enhance memory and agility, provide suppleness and strength to mind, enabling it to concentrate / meditate. All the mental faculties and systems get renewed energy, vigour. Higher values of mind are also aroused.

(9) They tone up the body, from top to bottom, regulate respiration, control cardiac, pulmonary, urinary and

digestive systems in such a perfect way that hardly any room is left for malfunctioning. They also purify and regulate circulation of blood, by fortifying lungs and heart.

(10) Each and every organ of the body is recharged and activated. Nervous system is toned up and diseases like hypertension, cardiac complications, mental tensions, stress, anger, agitation, approach to life are dispelled. In a way, where other therapies miserly fail and raise their hand up in digest and despair, yoga solves them in the shortest time and, above all, the sufferer feels relieved without any trace of side-effects.

(11) Those who practise the asanas regularly, improve their eyesight and, in certain cases, one may give up the use of aspects even or else his number may, at least, fall.

(12) Skin becomes soft , glossy, tender and strong enough to withstand thermic changes. Sudden weather changes have no or very little impact on the practice of Asanas.

(13) Facial wrinkles vanish, complexion, improves, signs of old age disappear and one feels to have gained a renewed vigour, vitality and glow. Rigid joints attain flexibility and mobility, especially flexibility of spine, which is necessary to retain and sustain youth. An old man even attains innocence and agility of a child.

(14) Asanas provide immunity against diseases, and also arouse prophylaxis.

(15) Other systems merely aim at toning up the body whereas yogasanas provide multifold benefits due to the fact that there are specific asanas for each and every disorder, whether physical or mental.

Importance of Yogic exercises as compared to other games/exercises

- Yogic exercises are very good for the exercise of internal organs of the body; like liver, pancreas, intestines, lungs, heart, kidneys, spine and joints etc. In other exercises– the internal organs are not exercised upto that level, as in Yogic exercises.

- In yoga the muscles are relaxed, heart beats are in perfect rhythm and the mind calm and peaceful as there is no competition while performing yoga, where as in sports, there is anxiety and stress due to competition.
- Yoga can be discontinued due to illness or certain other reasons with no side effects or weight gain, where as if games/other exercises are discontinued, there are chances of weight gain and lethargy.

Know about Precautions

- These exercises should not be performed by severely ill persons or who are bed ridden or suffering from acute slip disc pain or having a fracture.
- Females during pregnancy and menstruation should avoid and if required, perform only under supervision of an experienced yoga teacher.
- Children below the age of five years should not perform Yogic exercises, as there internal organs are very tender.
- If you are suffering from chronic ailments like arthritis, migraine, diabetes, renal failure, slip disc, cirrhosis of liver etc., perform these exercises only under supervision of a good yoga teacher.
- If you feel any pain during a particular exercise, stop doing that.
- If you feel exhausted, do 'Shavasana' at once, as this asana can be performed after any asana. Otherwise this particular asana is advised to be performed in last.

Factors Necessary for Performance of Yogasanas

Yoga is not exclusively meant for the benefits of saints, ascetics and mystics. It, in fact, serves to benefit all time taken to attain the desired result will depend on sincerity, regularity, patience and will to learn and perform. Burning desire to learn is the main driving force behind yoga, besides faith and confidence.

It is a complete, dependable and time-tested discipline and to derive optimum benefits, following points deserve to be borne in mind.

One should not nurture any ill-will, tension or inimical feeling. Apply yourself fully in the yogic sadhana and practice, forgetting worries and cares. Your mind should be in a happy and peaceful state, while you embark upon performing asanas. Try to overcome what ails you, physically and mentally.

Time

Ideal time to perform asanas is the early morning time, preferably sunset. Attend to the calls of nature and do not take anything before and after the exercises. If, however, morning time does not suit, asanas can be performed in the evening time also but on the premise that nothing should be taken 3-4 hours prior to performing yogic kriyas. While doing yoga do not exert undue strain on your limbs. Initially, due to lack of practice and rigidity of joints and muscles, it may take a bit longer time but, as the time passes, all such problems would disappear or, at best, show a declining trend for the better. Have patience; do not be cruel to your body as it will require some time to adjust itself to respond and withstand the demands made on it. It is not wise to change timings so be punctual and regular.

Place

Neat, clean, open, fresh environs are the prerequisites for yogic practice. Polluted, contaminated and unnatural environs will do more harm. If latter is the case, it is better to bid good-bye to such a practice, till such time as you are able to find suitable site. Open, green and clean gardens or countryside or bank or river are perhaps the most ideal places which are amiss in modern big cities. Instead, you can utilise your terrace for the purpose or else well ventilated rooms, where fresh air can enter without any disturbance. Proper place, light, open and fresh air, a soft blanket mat should always be handy. In winter you may use even a mattress or else a quilt may be used.

After competing an asana, give rest to your nerves, rather to whole body, and performing of shavasana (corpse posture / pose) would meet this requirement. Rest is necessary for the tired body and before you switch on to another asana, there should be a reasonable gap.

Rest

Whenever after doing an asana, you ever feel tired, at once suspend the asana and give proper rest to your body. Whenever, during course of an asana, you feel your body is getting tired and that you are unable to carry forward or continue any asana anymore, at once start relaxing your body. Fatigue is a warning signal from nature, warning you that as the optimum exertion has already of any consequence, what matters is how much mileage you have derived in the minimum of time span.

Bath

Bathing is not merely a ritual, it is also intended to purify the body. Bathing opens pores of the body also, when it is vigorously rubbed with a towel. If bath is taken before yoga postures, it would render the body light and also help on facilitating the process of asana. You can take bath with hot water, even after the asana is over, but a gap of 30 minutes is all the more necessary. Make sure that you towel your body in such a way that there is no moisture left on your body.

Dress

The dress used for the asanas should conform to weather conditions but, it must be ensured, that body is not overloaded with too much of clothes, as it will create problems while you are performing the asanas. Try to wear minimum of the clothes, but not so spared as to expose your body to ravages of atmosphere. Always wear loose clothes, as tight ones would restrict free movement of limbs. Ladies may use salwar-kameez or sacks and men underwears, trousers or half pants for the performance of asanas.

Breakfast

There should ideally be a gap of half-an-hour between asanas and breakfast. Take only light and easily digestible breakfast and should not be so much to fill your belly to the full. Avoid taking any cold drink or food immediately after an asana is over. If you wish, you may have a glassful of milk (Hot).

Sun-Bath

It will always be handy. In winter you may use even a mattress or else a quilt may be used.

General

All the asanas are based on and named after parts of the body, material objects, and animals. There are innumerable asanas but, in practice only 84 asanas are said to meet all the disorders which afflict all persons, in one way, or at one time or the other. Asanas are not medicines or tonics, they tend to correct the wrongs done by us. They also awaken our auto-immune mechanism which is adversely affected by various factors. They correct the defective metabolism, inducing and fortifying the fighting capacity of our body to drive out the invading forces. They aim at rooting out the cause of the malady which often emanates from disturbance of the mind.

❑

32

YOGASANAS FOR REIKI PRACTITIONERS

There are some yogasanas also which have to be performed with the practice of Pranayama.

Padmasana (Lotus Pose)

Method: It is called Padmasana because while performing it, legs appear in the form of a lotus. Sit on the ground and stretch forward your legs, keeping them together. Now left foot should be placed over the right thigh, and right foot over the left thigh, making sure that the heels touch the abdomen on both sides on the either side of nail. Keep the hands on the knees. Keep the head and back portion erect. Both the feet should touch the ground, and eyes be kept closed. This asana can be utilised for doing Pranayama. If you wish, you can join index finger and thumbs, base of thumb resting on index finger's nail, a Sign of Mudra Pranayama.

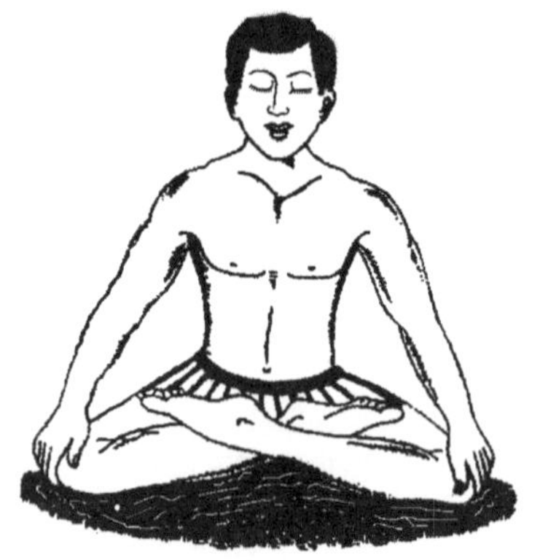

Padmasana

Benefits: It is very useful to gain concentration of mind, to enhance mental faculties, to do mental work, especially useful for the aged person. It prevents trapping of wind in the body; preserves vital fluids of the body, imparts solace, peace, solitude and longevity. It tones up reproductive organs and system of females, prevents and cures abdominal disorders. For dhyana (meditation), padmasana is unique and ideal asana.

Sarvangasana (Pan Physical Pose)

Method: Lie flat on the ground, your spine touching the floor, stretch the body raise the legs slowly and let them stay at right angle to the trunk. After staying for a few seconds slowly raise up the body, without giving any jerk to the spine. Take help from the hands, keeping the fingers outward and thumbs towards the belly. Slowly go on raising the back until the whole trunk is at 90^0 and the entire weight comes on the shoulders and neck. Take the legs slightly forward and press the chest with your chin. After remaining in the said pose for a few seconds come to the original position.

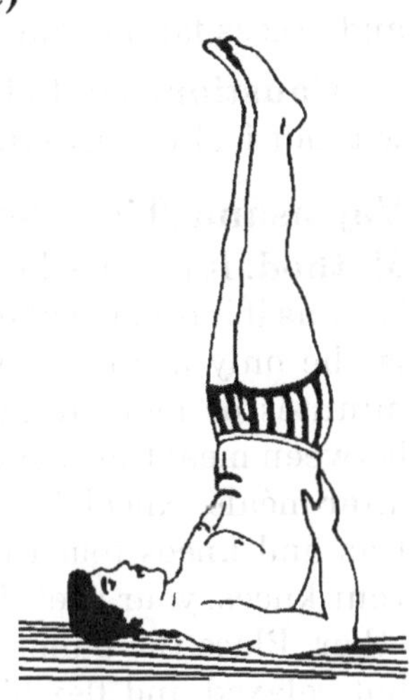
Sarvangasana

Benefits: This asana cures constipation, dyspepsia, has a salutary effect on thyroid gland, tones up the nervous system, all limbs of the body, helps to preserve and thicken semen, is useful in intestinal disorders, varicose veins, appendicitis, renders spine flexible, throat disorders are removed, gas is expelled. In addition, it gives glow, vitality and strength to the body, increases sex power, removes menstrual disorders. Persons with hypertension and cordial problems should never take to this asana, except under advice and guidance and supervision of a yoga teacher.

Halasana

Method: Half of this asana is same as you have done in Sarvangasana. You have too bend your legs behind your head and in doing this your head and knees should not bend.

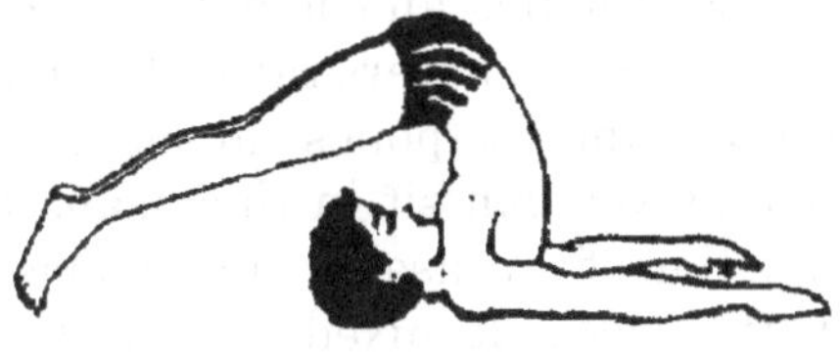
Halasana

Benefits: This is very good asana to cure digestive disorders and access fat on your abdomen.

Caustion: Try to bend you legs as much as you can bend without feeling any strain and slowly try to touch the ground.

Vajrasana (Thunderbolt Posture)

Method: It is named thunderbolt, as it imparts the strength to body as if it is made like a stone or as strong as a thunder bolt. It is the only asana, in yoga, which can be practised after 45 minutes or more from the time of finishing your meals. In between meal times, it can also be done, but never immediately after meals. Kneel down on the floor, letting your big toes, and legs and knees touch the ground. Now rest your buttocks on your knees, your heels bent inwards and thumbs touching each other. Place the palms on the knees, keeping your spine erect but relaxed and flexible. Breathing should be even, deep and slow. Expand your chest, drawing the abdominal muscles inwards.

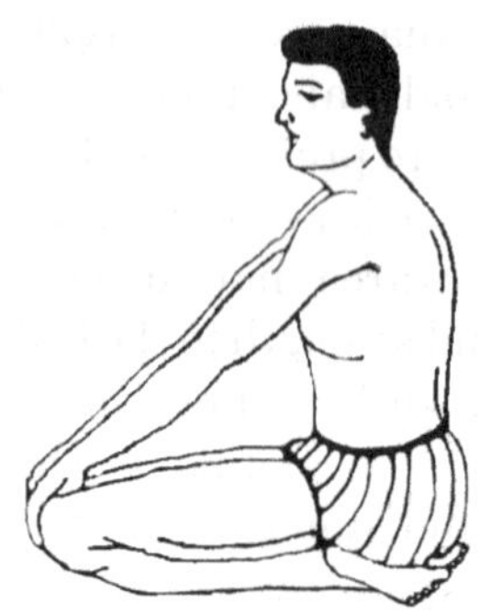

Vajrasana

Benefits: This asana will expel gas and remove acidity. How much you have overeating, it will digest the same. It tones up sexual system of both males and females, removes pain and stiffness in spine and knees, lowers raised blood pressure, gives longevity and retards and postpones old age. For meditation, it is an ideal asana, as you can sit in this asana as long as you wish. After completion of this asana, simply massage with your hands or, still better, use salt mixed oil, say of mustard, which can be slightly Luke-warmed.

Bhujang or Sarpasana (Cobra /Serpent Pose)

Method: Lie flat on the ground, abdominal portion touching the ground. Straighten both the arms, palms touching the ground. Now bring the palms at level with both sides of abdomen. Slowly lift your neck and torso in such a way that whole body rests on your palms. Now lift your neck upwards gradually and try to look upwards as far and as conveniently you can. Let the toes touch the ground and palms securely resting on the ground. Do not let your elbows bend down. Stay in the position as long you can. When you feel suffocated or when there is a feeling that you can't endure / continue any more, then slowly get back to original position from where you had started. After the asana is over, loosen your limbs and relax.

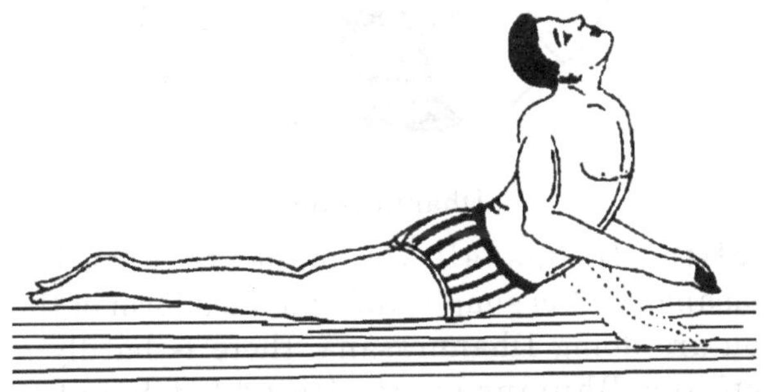

Bhujang or Sarpasana

Benefits: Abdominal muscles and back portion are supplied with blood and blood circulation in general, is improved and also fresh and pure blood is supplied to all the organs. It imparts strength, flexibility and tone to spinal column. It removes menstrual disorders and irregularity, helps to improve digestion, chance of night discharge is dispelled, helps to maintain celibacy. It is useful for diabetics, as it activates the pancreas, thereby causing secretion of insulin, render arms, hands and neck painless, flexible and active. Kidneys and intestines also are strengthened. It removes obesity and sheds extra flesh from the abdominal portion, and spinal curvature and postural abnormalities are also removed.

Dhanurasana (Bow-Shaped Posture)

Method: Lie flat on the ground, your abdominal side touching the ground. Fold your legs from the knees. Now lift your neck and torso, gradually keeping your hands along sides of your back. Try to catch hold of your ankles with your hands. Gradually stretch your hands and feet so that they form a bow-shape, stay in this position as long as you can. Then regain the former position and relax by loosening your limbs.

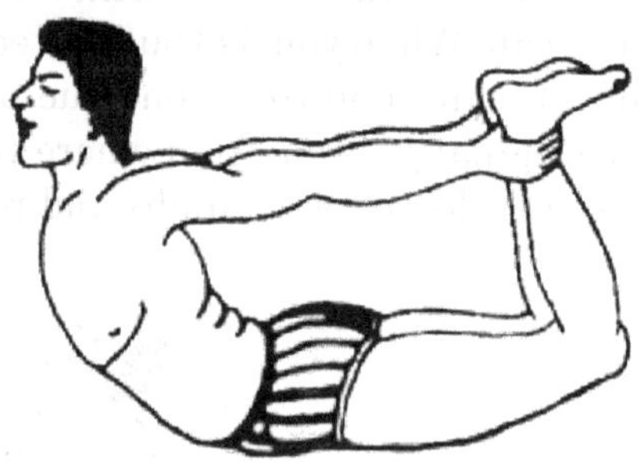

Dhanurasana

Benefits: It has all the benefits detailed under Bhujangasana, as it is simply and extended form of the former. When you are doing Dhanurasana, there is hardly any need for practising Bhujangasana. Its added benefits are in strengthening of hands, elbows, ankles, knees. In short, both the lower and upper extremities become more flexible and strong, abdominal pressure helps in secretion of digestive juice and activities endocrine glands. In both these asanas, no jerk should be exerted on any organ. This suggestion is good for all other asanas too. Pregnant ladies must not perform this asana.

Gomukhasana (The Cow-Face Posture)

Method: Sit on the floor, keeping the legs stretched forward. Fold the left leg at the knee and sit on the left foot with the help of hands, fold the right leg and place the right thigh on the left thigh. Bring heels of both the feet together so that they touch each other which can be done by lifting your buttocks a bit. Now bend your right arm from the ear (right side) and bring the hand on the back side of your end. Fold the left hand behind your back and try to form a hook in which both the hands are clasped. Care should be taken not to over exert your limbs. Gradually you will get to the desired position as your limbs attain flexibility. Keep yourself in this position for about 30 seconds. Thereafter, give yourself some pause and reverse the position of hands and legs. If a lady wishes to develop her breast on a particular side, she should perform this asana more with the hand of that side (on which she wishes to develop her breast).

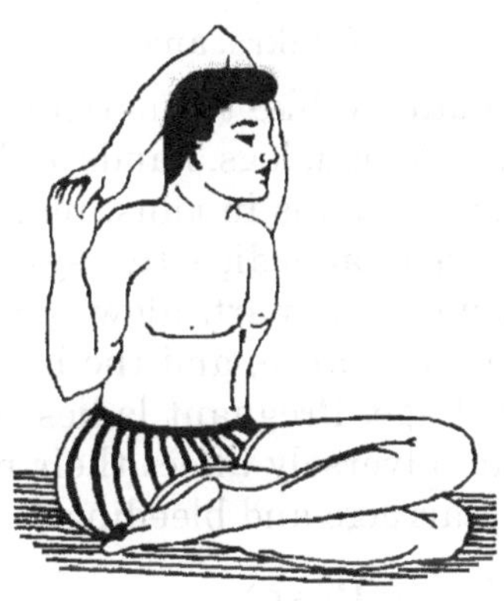

Gomukhasana

Benefits: This asana is equally beneficial for both the males and females, as it strengthens the muscle of shoulder, chest / breast and makes legs stronger. Muscles of relevant organs are also rendered elastic. After completing the asana, whether on either or both sides, never strain your limbs. Initially, you may find it convenient to perform the asana on one side only, but regular practice will remove all the hesitancy and stiffness, thus making way for you to do the asana on the other side too.

Chakrasana (A Circle Pose)

Method: On a hard surface, lie flat on your back. Later, raise the middle portion of your body upwards, fixing and keeping firmly both the feet and hands on the ground thus making a semi-circle, ensuring that your head keeps between your hands. Now concentrate your eyes on something that lies in front of you.

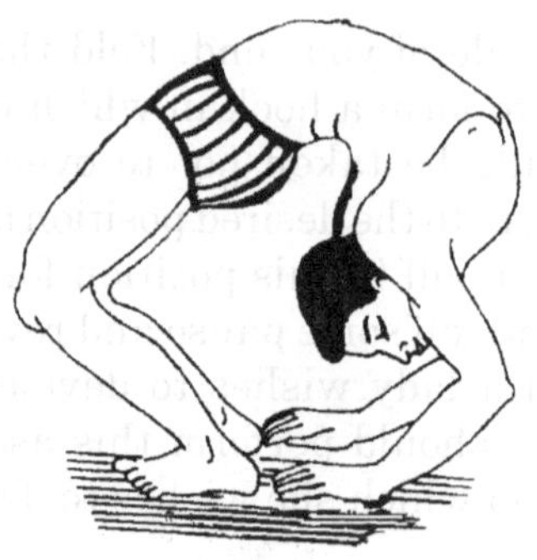

Chakrasana

Benefits: It enhances, like the sarvangasana, strength of head, throat, neck, abdomen, legs, hands and, in short, all parts of your body, eliminates pains in joins, removes extra fat from the abdominal area, activates digestive system, renders spinal column elastic and supple, imparts glow and agility to the body, normalises posture and stance, and the body stays erect even during the advanced age. Pregnant ladies should not practice this asana as it can adversely affect their pregnancy process, even leading to miscarriage and bleeding.

Kagasana (The Crow Pose)

Method: This asana can be done 3 or more times in a day at the rate of 30 seconds per asana or more. Squat on the floor. Keep the arms between your heels and legs, heels being raised on toes. Now, place both the palms flat on the ground (in front), while keeping arms in line and shoulders stretched out as much as possible. Thereafter, raise your body on the toes and endeavour to put pressure on your already spread hands. Remain in this position from ½ to 1 minute and then retrace to the original position and finally relax.

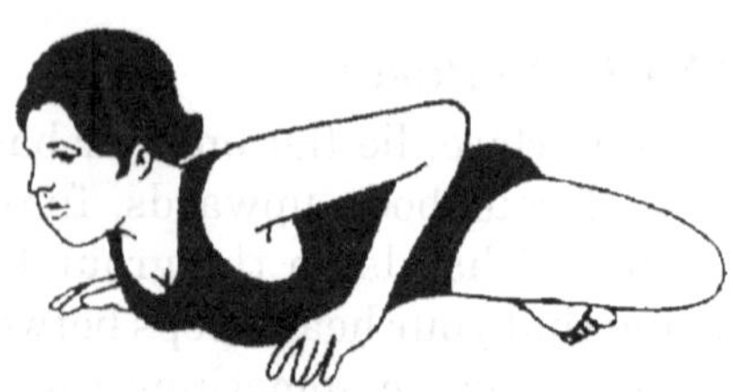

Kangasana

Benefits: This posture helps to diminish the unwanted arches on the spine by helping it to elongate, it strengthens muscles of arms and shoulders, helps to activate hormonal secretions. Old, emaciated and pregnant ladies should resist from doing this asana. Those who have pains in arms, hands and fingers should also abstain, as weak limbs may not be able to withstand weight of the body. This asana should be practised, like many other asanas, on empty stomach only.

Kukkutasana (Cock Pose)

Method: Sit in the position of Padamasana. Insert the hands between the opening to thighs and calves. Now push down the hands and plant them firmly on the floor, keeping your fingers fully spread. Now, after that, push the legs and thighs up your arms. In doing so, your hands turn full so that you could exert desired and sustainable force in lifting the body up. Keep your torso in and upright position, as far as possible. Remain in the final position for a minute or so.

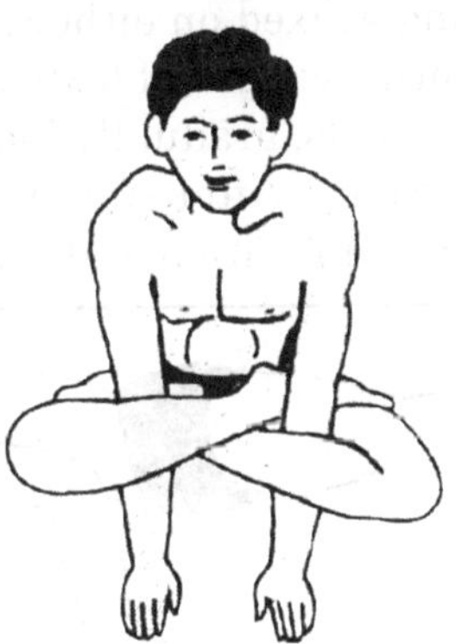

Kukkutasana

Benefits: Your chest and shoulder muscles become firm due to pressure on them. It also develops and hardens breast-line of females who have small breasts, provided they practise this posture for quite some time.

Mahavirasana (Named after Lord Mahavir/Hanuman)

Method: Stand erect, bringing forward one foot to a distance of 3 feet from the other. Clench fists of both the hands and raise them. Now, go on jumping alternatively on both the feet, changing the pressure on each feet alternatively. Keep your lips to each other and breath through nose only. When you are tired, take pause until you regain strength to resume the asana. Loosen your limbs and relax.

Benefits: It increases height, sheds extra weight from the waist, body is rendered stronger, chest expands, legs, arms and feet gain strength. It increases sexual power, especially of men, restores normally to menstrual cycle.

Mayurasana (Peacock Pose)

Method: Stand erect alongside of a table. Place both the hands firmly on top of the table. Fold your both elbows in such a way that the elbows touch and remain firmly (touched) near naval. Now, exert whole weight on your hands, by lifting your body at 180^0 and try to stay in this position for 40-50 seconds, increasing the duration gradually or, alternatively, spread some blanket or still better lie flat on ground. Firmly affix your hands on ground, your elbows remaining affixed on either side of navel. Now lift your body and put entire weight of body on the hands. Stay in that position for 40 seconds, gradually increasing the duration, depending on your capacity. After staying in that position, very slowly regain the original position and relax.

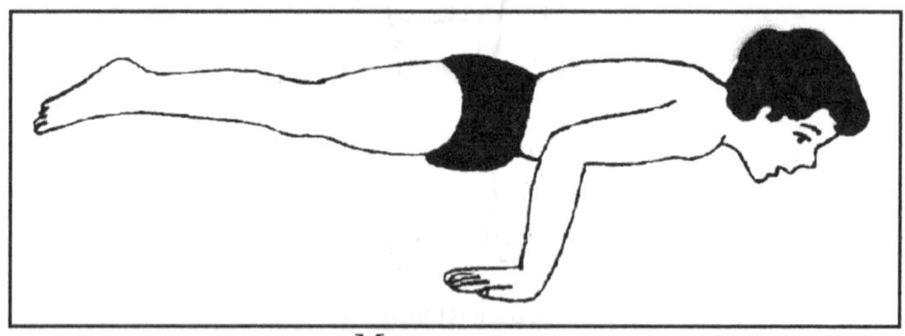

Mayurasana

Benefits: Increases digestion and appetite. Intestines gain strength, constipation and indigestion are dispelled. Liver and kidney disorders get relieved. Above all, if you have taken poison or poisonous food, it will remove the poison and its effects. It is well known that the snake is eaten by the peacock and its name justifies its utility, as it helps to strengthen the body. Pregnant ladies must not do this asana.

Note: Maximum benefits from the said and other asanas can be derived only when performed properly without exceeding your physical capacity, keeping in view your state of health. To derive optimum benefits, to cure a particular disease or disorder, precision and correctness with which an asana is performed and whether all the relevant procedures have been complied with, are the factors which can ensure utility of an asana.

To start with, proper guidance, or how, what and where of each asana intended to be performed should be guided by a yoga teacher and his guidance sought, if and when some problem is encountered. Never exert undue strain on your body because all asanas cannot be performed by all persons and also all asanas are not required to be done by all. Books on yoga, however precise and meticulous they may be, will only give you an initial motivation in the form of a launching pad only. Without a guru, knowledge gained remains half-baked, hence do not forget what you are expected to do and what not.

Parvatasana

Sit in Padmasana (that is by keeping left foot on the right thigh and right foot on the left thigh). Inhale breath and raise both the hands towards the sky, keeping all the fingers apart and stretching both arms without bending either of them. Stay in the said position as per your capacity and convenience but do not overdo. Before you get suffocated, gradually bring down both the arms and place on both the knees and relax, but without binding your back. Keep spinal column erect at 90°. The process can be repeated a number of times. In normal conditions ladies can also perform this asana, but never during pregnancy.

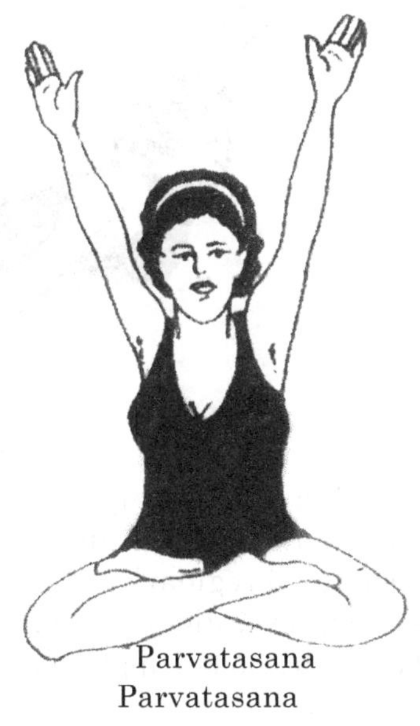

Parvatasana

Parvatasana

This asana imparts flexibility to the spine, strengthens arms, expands chest, and adds to strength of arms and fingers. Improves flexibility of shoulder blades. It improves upon asthmatic condition and tones up uterus.

Yanasana

While performing this asana, body assumes shape and form of a plane flying in the sky; here its nomeclation as such.

Life flats on the floor, while your abdomen touches the ground. Keep both the feet touching each other. First inhale and then raise your head, neck, hands, chest and feet above the ground, keeping all these organs tight and straight-only your abdomen touching the ground. When you feel you cannot retain the inhaled breath. Relax and loosen your limbs. After sometime, it can be repeated 3-4 times or even more, if capacity permits. Even while maintaining normal breath, this asana can also be performed. Pregnant women must never perform this asana.

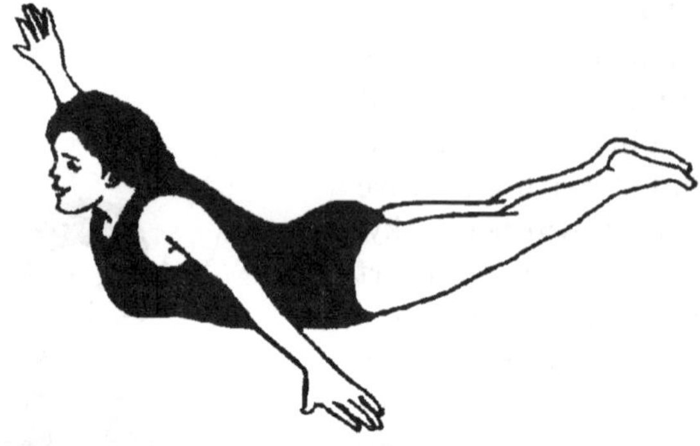

Yanasana

This asana helps to strengthen bones of arms, hands, shoulders, and legs and also imparts flexibility to the spine. If performed regularly, it can add to inches also. It removes extra fat, improves digestion, removes almost all uterine disorders, and keeps the body supple. This asana is not suitable for pregnant ladies.

Stand erect and keep the feet apart at a distance of 6" to lift. Now gradually bring down the hands and try to touch the ground in front of your toes. While doing so, exert no pressure nor strain unduly. If initially you cannot touch the ground, it is advisable to bend only to the extent possible. As your back and spine become supple, process will look much easier. Do not bend knees, and elbows, keeping your neck straight at 180° while your eyes are affixed looking at the ground or at your hands.

This asana elongates legs and arms, makes spine flexible and supple, improves eyesight, strengthens bones and muscles of legs and hands, and does away with trembling. Persons with backache, hip-joint disease and pregnant ladies must not perform this asana. It also strengths heart, improves cardiac output and efficiency. Improves respiration.

Note: As a general rule any forward bending asana or any physical exercise should never be performed by persons having stiff back, backache and lumbar/spinal spondylysis/curvature. Backward bending asana/exercise may be performed if advised by the concerned experts.

Matsyasana

Sit in Padmasana and thereafter lie down on your back. Catch hold of big toe of feet with hands and rise up your back portion in a gradual manner. In this position your backside of head and knees should knees should continue to touch the ground. Retain breath as long you can and stay in the final position and exhale while returning to the previous state.

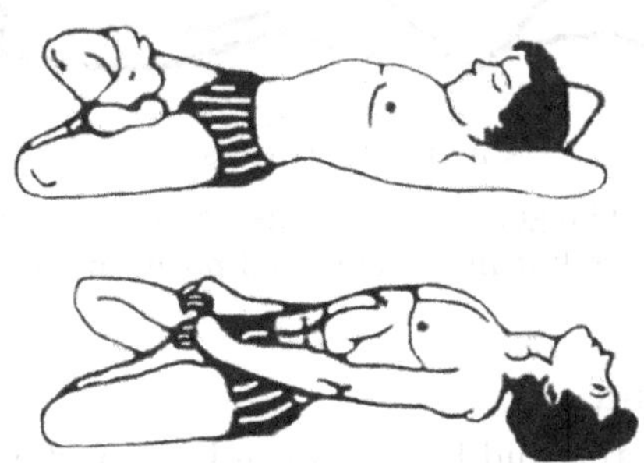

Matsyasana

It strengthens chest and lungs, removes extra fat from hips, strengthens legs and hands, dispels asthma, and removes constipation and also column also ensured. In normal health conditions ladies can perform this asana, but not during pregnancy.

Pashchimottanasana

Sit on the floor and spread both legs in front of you and each hold of your big toes with both the hands, but do not let your knees bend. In order to catch the toes you have to bend the back. Initially it may seem slightly difficult to do so, due to rigidity of muscles and limbs; hence do not exert but gradually posture. In 4-5 sitting your body will get attuned to the final posture. Persons with back pain and stiff and muscles, pregnant ladies should not perform this asana unless and until advised by a doctor or yoga expert.

It strengthens legs, arms and renders the spine flexible and supple, improve digestion, removes fat on and around abdomen, constipation fortifies and rejuvenates energy and nervous system, lengthens leg bones, Purifies blood, improves liver, cardiac and respiratory processes, removes fat from hips and sideways.

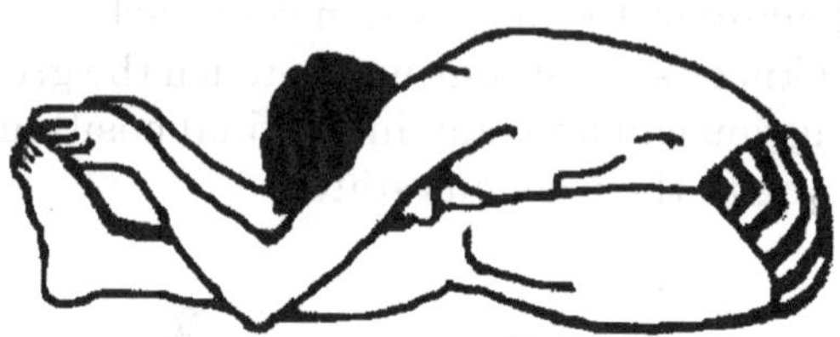

Pashchimottanasana

Note: Those who get adept on this asana, may try to touch their knees with the nose but in the changed position also knees shouldn't be bent.

Janushirasana

Sit on the floor and fold leg from the knee and place heel of left leg below the anus. Keeping the other leg straight. Catch hold of the right foot and try to touch the knee of the speed out leg with your nose/ mouth. There won't be any difficulty if you can

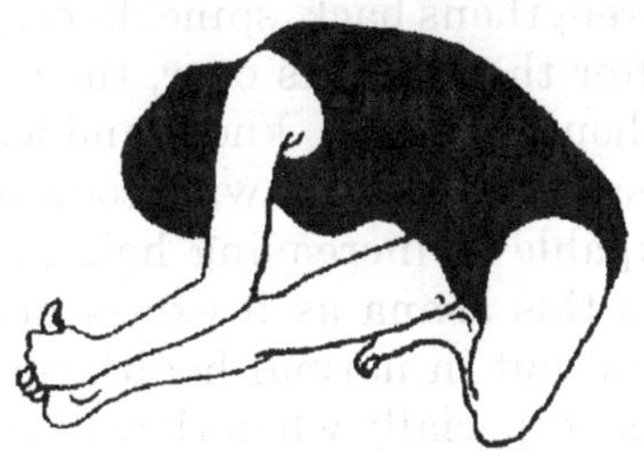

Janushirasana

perform the 'Pashchimottana Asana'. Return to normal position. Now repeat the same process with the right leg. When done, relax. You may fully succeed after 5-6 attempts and until a successful posture is achieved never exert undue pressure. Pregnant ladies, backache persons who have stiff spine, muscles and joints, should not perform it, but others may proceed gradually in a phased manner.

Ushtrasana

This asana has been named after the camel.

Sit erect and let the weight of entire body fall on both knees and toes of feet. Now catch hold of your heels with the hands, as shown in the figure. While performing this asana, make sure that the back is bent in such a way that neck bends towards feet, back also bends slightly. Look upwards. Stay in the final position as far and as you conveniently can. Retain breath and exhale while getting back to the original (starting) position.

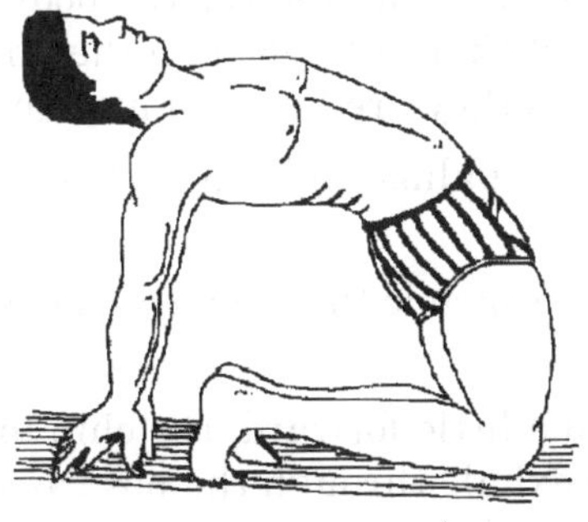

Ushtrasana

This asana strengthens back, spine, knees, and feet renders spine flexible. After the asana is over, there may be felt ache and stiffness in shoulder blades, knees and feet. To ward off all such effects massage these parts with coconut or mustard oil. This asana is capable of increasing height. Pregnant ladies shouldn't perform this asana as it exerts utmost pressure on abdomen and back, but in normal health condition, they may perform this asana, especially when they have backache. Avoid undue pressure and jerk in any case.

Sinhamudra

Yogic exercises should accompany breathing in rhythm only through the nostrils. This asana is an exception where one cannot do so, because the tongue has to be folded and then stretched in two stages.

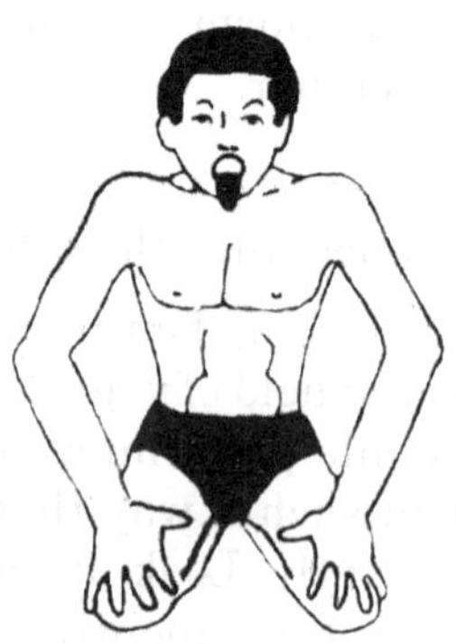

Sinhamudra

Method: Kneel down and lower the body to sit on heels as in Vajrasana except that in Vajrasana the knees are kept close together and in this they are kept slightly apart.

Spread both the palms and place them on the knees in a relaxed way.

Breath evenly, protrude the tongue and fold inwards to touch the palate.

Bend the head a little forward, the chin touching the chest. At the same time exhale through the nose as well as the mouth simultaneously stretching the tongue as much as possible out of the mouth.

Widen the eyes and fix the gaze in front.

Remain thus for two-three seconds and not more during the initial days.

Once the protrusion of the tongue is completed, you should stop exhaling and hold the breath for two seconds. After two seconds, slowly draw in the tongue and inhale only through the nose and sit erect.

Repeat the process again. After a few days of practice, this exercise can be perfected and practised as many times as possible.

Benefits: This exercise is extremely useful to all young children and must be practised by adults to prevent and cure a number of diseases connected with ear, nose, throat and other respiratory troubles.

It helps greatly in overcoming all problems related to tonsils, adenoids, larynx and pharynx. If regularly practised, it can prevent any unnecessary removal of tonsils by surgery. As the face and eye muscles are exercised, it gives a glowing colour to the complexion and shine to the eyes. This exercise proves to be extremely beneficial to singers and public speakers. It is useful in all forms of skin diseases. It cures thyroid diseases and deafness if practised perfectly and regularly.

Mandukasana

This asana must have derived its name for the Sanskrit name Manduka which means a frog. Mandukasana does not resemble the frog very much as its name denotes, but the folded legs resemble frog's hind legs and the arms supporting the body look like frog's forelegs. Though this asana looks simple and is also easy to perform, its benefits are plenty.

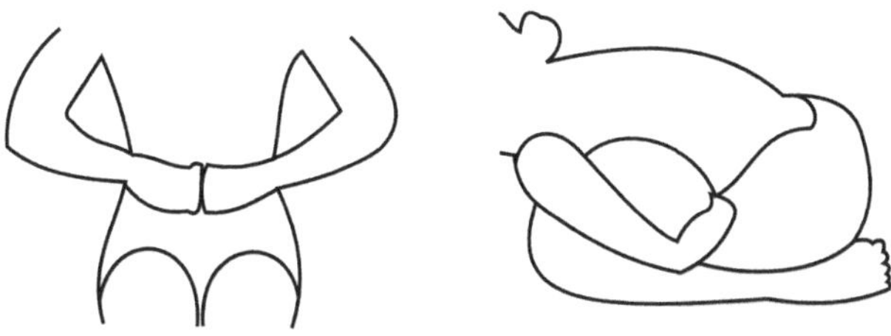

Mandukasana

Method: Kneel down with the knees apart.

Slowly lower the body and sit down between the folded legs in such a way that the buttocks touch the ground. Slowly widen the gap between the knees till they come in a straight line.

Keep the toes close to each other. Lean a little forward and place both the palms near the thighs, fingers turned towards the thighs.

Keep the spine erect, fix your gaze straight and breath normally. Stay so for as long as you can and revert back to original position by releasing the hands first and then drawing in the folded legs together.

Relax and repeat again.

During the initial days of practice, difficulty may be experienced in spreading the legs and it may not come in straight line. The groins may ache if you force it. Gradually, the gap can be decreased without any discomfort.

Benefits: This is a unique exercises for women, teenage girls as well as women of other ages.

All uttering disorders respond well to this exercise. The so-called premenstrual syndrome, like depression, frustration and anxiety can be overcome by practising this asana regularly.

It cures impotence in the males. It strengthens the pelvic muscles and improves circulation in the region.

It helps control bladder and prostate disorders.

Spinal nerves get adequate supply of circulation and they become stronger.

It is a good exercise for obesity too.

❑

33
RELAXATION EXERCISES

Shavasana (Yoganidra)

Lie down straight with your back on the ground. Keep a distance of one foot between the legs and keeping both the hands little further from the thighs, keep the hands slightly open towards upward direction. Close the eyes, neck straight, the whole body should be relaxed. Slowly take four to five deep breaths and leave. Now, look at each part of the body through your mind with determination and experience that each organ is in relaxed condition and tension free. Determination is the force behind all the works and great objectives. Now we have to give complete rest to our body. For this also we have to take the determination of relaxing and resting the body.

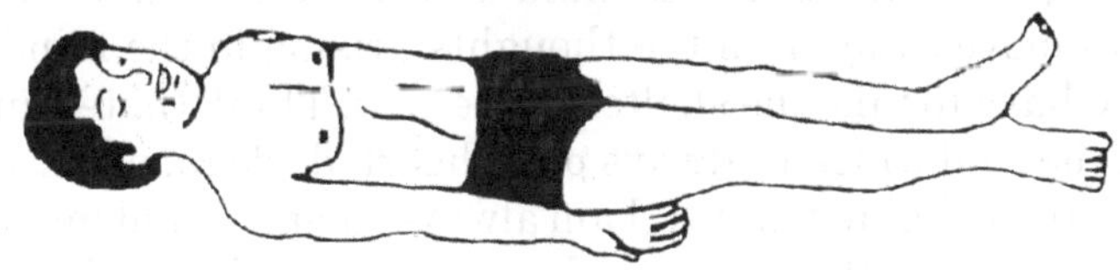

Shavasana

First and foremost, with the determination of the mind look at the toes of legs leave them totally loose and tension free. After toes look at the ankles experience their relaxation. Now see the calf muscles and think that my calf muscles are absolutely healthy, tension free and in the position of total rest and experience that the whole body is getting rest by the mere feeling of relaxation. As we start crying with the feeling of extreme sorrow, we laugh with the feeling of happiness, and the blood starts boiling with the mere feeling of victory, in the same way the body starts experiencing total rest only with the mere feeling of relaxation. After calf muscles now looking at the knees, experience that they are healthy, and in the condition of tension free. Within the mind look at the thighs and experience them to be in the condition of total rest. After thighs gradually look at the upper parts of the body-waist, stomach, back, looking at them with ease experience the situation of total rest, health and tension free. Now with quiet feeling concentrate the mind on the heart and try to listen to the heart beats. Listen to the divine tune of the heart and think that my heart is absolutely heatlhy, tension free and in the situation of total rest, there is no disorder or disease in my heart. Now relaxing the lungs and the heart, look at the shoulders and experience them to be in the situation of tension free and totally relaxed. Then look at hands, elbows, wrists and fingers of both the hands and big fingers and experience the hands to be in the situation of tension free, relaxed, and total rest.

Now look at the face and think there is no worry, tension, disappointment or any negative feeling on my face. There is happiness, gladness, expectation and calmness on my face. There is unlimited happiness on my face including my eyes, nose, ears. Till now we have given to give total rest to the body with the nave to give total rest to the mind and relax the Mind. Now we have to move away from the thoughts arising in the mind. For this we have to take the shelter of the soul. Think that–I am the son of the soul which is always pure-hearted, clean, pious, clam, happy, and enlighten nectar. I am always complete and immortal. I do not lack anything, in fact I am always full of feelings and devotion. I am the part of the happy form of the God. I am the nectar son of the God. I am separate from the bonds of nature, body, senses and mind. My natural shelter is my God. I do not become popper, poor, orphan or possessing a parent or guardian or a king with the increase and decrease of outside prosperity. I am always one essence. The changes which are taking place are the duties of the world, my soul has no duties. In this way think about the divinity of the soul and remove the negative thinking, because negative thinking makes a person sad, worried, and stressed. Negative thinking makes a person depressed and always immersed in the ocean of grief. Positive thinking person is always happy, normal, and cheerful even in the adverse situations. For this reason, the person should have positive thinking not only at the time of yoganidra or Shavasan but during the whole day. In this way we have thought positive about the divine form of the soul and gave rest to the mind and now we will think about the divine form of the God and give total rest to our soul.

Think that your soul has come out of the body and it is lying above the body in the sky and you are experiencing with the internal soul that the body is lying on the ground just like a dead body. This is the reason that this asana is called Shavasan. Now devote your conscious strength to the God who is spread in the unending sky in the form of Supreme Soul Brahma. Think that your soul is the divine happiness of the God from all sides. Experience the divine happiness of the God's creation. The determination which is auspicious and with completed devotion towards God, is complete. You think of this God's nature and its divinity and concentrating on the wonderful form and creation of nature think of God's divinity. Think that you are in the valley of beautiful flowers, and the whole atmosphere is full of the scent of the different kinds of beautiful flowers. There is a kind of divinity on all sides. It is a great sight to see the God's creation. There is no cnd to God's creation. Along with the flowers plants, there are beautiful fruits on the different trees, the God has filled each fruit with different flavours. A light breeze is flowing from all sides and giving immense happiness. In this beautiful garden the birds are chirping the divine songs of the God's creation. One can see God appearing from each flower, fruit. When we look at the sky it appears that the stars, the Moon and the Sun are like diyas in the huge universe in the form of temple. The rivers are flowing as if they are washing the feet of the God. Brahma is so great, unlimited, unbounded, unending. Oh God! Oh Father! Creator of the earth, Oh Mother! Take your son also in yoru shelter. Bless me with your divine happiness. Oh Lord! I should always get your divinity, calmness and enlightment. I should always remember your divine creations and immerse in your, and be engrossed in the unending happiness. Oh God! take me out of the wordly feelings and take me in the lap of happiness.

In this way take the incomparable happiness and once again experience yourself in the body. Imagine that you have returned back to the body after full sleep of Yoga. The respiration is on. Along with the breath the great power of life source is entering inside you. Experience yourself to be healthy, happy and cheerful and in the way the body was relaxed with determination in the same way and with the same determination experience the new power, consciousness and happiness in the body. Look at each organ from toe to the head and whichever organ you are seeing imagine that it is absolutely healthy. For example, if a person has pain in the knee or backache he should imagine that his pain has been relieved. By God's grace and practice of Yoga there is no pain in my knees and back, because Yoga cures the root cause of these diseases. The pain is coming out. In the same way there is any heart or stomach problem think that it has been cured. If there is any blockage in the arteries and the cholesterol level is high then think that the diseases are being cured. Take the vow that all the foreign particles, diseases, and deformities are going out and I am totally healthy. With these thoughts you should experience yourself to be physically and mentally healthy.

In the end experience that both the hands are totally powerful and healthy and rub both the palms against each other and keep the warm palms on your eyes and slowly open the eyes. This is the summarized method of Yoganidra and Shavasan. If anybody is unable to sleep then before going to bed, practice Shavasan and relax the body and feel tension free in the directed method and think of God's divinity and concentrate on the respiration and with every breath chant Omkar in the mind. While inhaling and exhaling meaningful chanting of Omkar should be done. The meaning of Omkar is Brahma in the form of God, Omkar God is always in the form of truth, consciousness and cheerful. I am also getting happiness by praying the Omkar God. With these thoughts one should chant Omkar. The speed of inhaling and exhaling should be normal. In the same process count reverse from 100 to 1 and with each number chant Om. For example, Om 10, Om 99, Om 98 etc. Praying in this way will put you off to deep sleep and you will get rid of bad dreams. In the daily yoga practice, this asana should be done after every difficult asana. After the end of practice, this asana should be done for 5 to 10 minutes.

Benefits:

1. Mental stress, depression, high blood pressure, heart disease and insomnia are cured. These patients should do this asana regularly.
2. Weakness of the nervous system, tiredness, negative thinking are cured.
3. The body, mind, brain and soul gets total rest, power, zeal and happiness.
4. The concentration power increases.
5. Practicing Shavasan in between asanas relieves the tiredness of the body.

Makarasan

Process

1. Lie straight with your stomach towards the ground. While folding both the hands keep them on the opposite shoulders.
2. Rest the forehead on the hands. There should be one foot distance between the legs.
3. Relax the body like a dead body. While lying down in this position think of a dead body and concentrate yourself within the soul through wise thinking and introspection. I am a separate life, pure-hearted and cheerful and flawless soul . This body is perishable. This body is the collection of five elements. When the time comes it merges in the same elements. This body and other riches remain here. We do not bring anything with us neither we will take anything along. In this way deviate your mind from the mortal world and experience the happiness of devotion to the Brahma present in the unending universe.

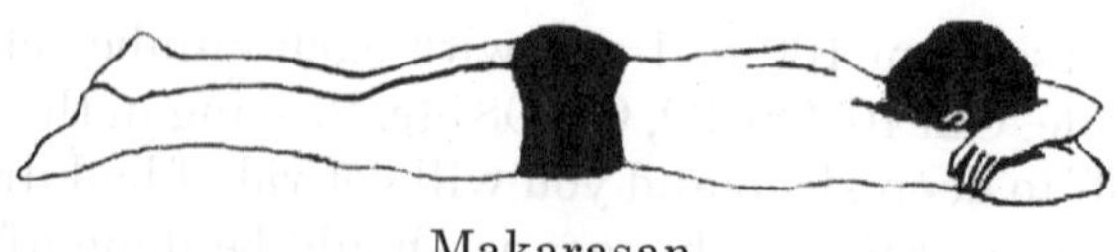

Makarasan

Benefits

1. This is the asana for rest. During rest a person feels light not only physically but also mentally. He is free from high blood pressure, mental tension and insomnia. In-between the asana this should be done for rest. The intestines of the stomach get natural massage which activates them and dysentery and other deformities are cured.
2. Since the hands are in passive stretching condition it affects the sympathetic nerves and helps in the relaxation of the body.
3. The heart does not function against the magnetic force, therefore it gets rest.
4. The internal secretion glands are benefited.

Balasan (Rest Position)

Process

1. Lie down with your stomach towards the ground keep the left hand under the head on the ground and turning the neck to the right keep the head on the hands, the left hand will be under the head and the left palm will be under the right hand.
2. Fold the right knee slightly, the way a child sleeps, lie down like that and rest. In the same way this asana is done from the other side.

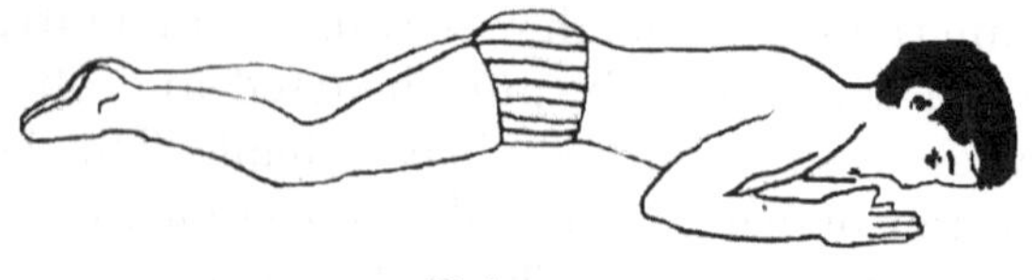

Balasan

Benefits

Just like Shavasan, the tiredness of the body and mind is relieved.

❑

34

SHAT KARM: SIX YOGIC KRIYAS

These Yogic Kriyas are the purification processes of the body by yogic methods. They are very important in Yoga. Union of body with mind, union of mind with soul and union of soul with God is Yoga.

Kriyas are to be practised early in the morning before sunrise on empty stomach. Kriyas must be finished before starting the Asanas or Pranayama.

These Kriyas consist of six purification practises:

1. Dhauti (Kunjal)
2. Basti
3. Neti
4. Tratak
5. Nauli, and
6. Kapalbhati.

Dhauti (Kunjal)

Vomit-Dhauti-Cleaning. Washing stomach by water.

Two or three litre of tepid water is required. Squat on your feet back, spine and neck should be straight. Drink glasses of tepid water continuously without any pause upto the brim of neck. One should neither talk nor laugh during this period. He should not bend and should stand.

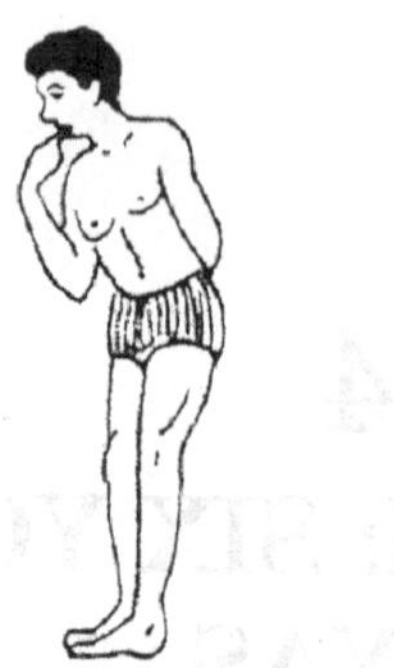
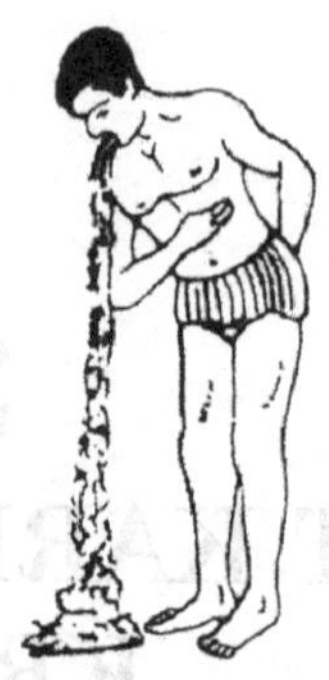

Dhauti

Bend a bit forward. Keep the left hand on the left knee and the first and second finger of the right hand in your throat. Press the stomach by the other hand. You will vomit. Vomit the whole drunk water. Water should not remain in stomach.

Wash you hands and take rest. Milk or breakfast should be taken after an hour.

This Dhauti kriya should be practised after passing stool and after bath. One should not take bath after this kriya. Vaman Dhauti kriya should be practised once a fortnight or once a month.

Precautions: 1. Heart patients should not practise it. 2. The nails of the fingers should be trimmed otherwise they may wound the throat.

Benefits: 1. Disorders of bile and gas are cured. 2. It is beneficial in the diseases of stomach throat and jaundice.

Basti (Enema)

Enema pot, rubber tube, nozzle, tepid water, lemon are the requirements. Mix juice of one or two lemons in the tepid water. Fill the enema pot with water.

Suspend the enema pot one metre above. Apply a little oil or vaseline to the nozzle of the rectal tube. Before insertion, check the rectal tube to ensure free flow of water. Insert the tube into the rectum. The flow of water can be adjusted with the knob attached to the tube. When all the water has been introduced,

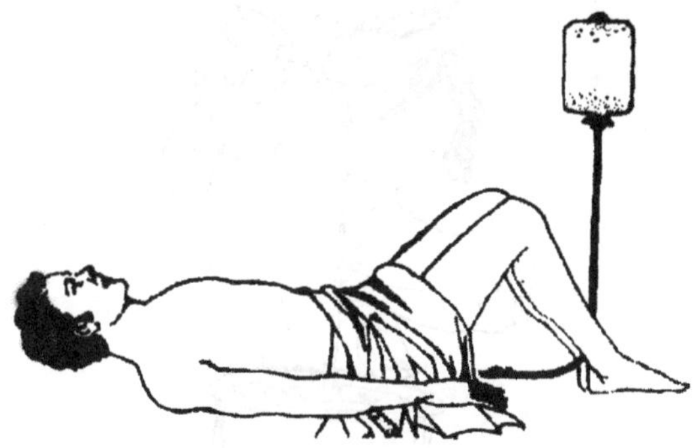

Basti (Enema)

remove the tube and resist the pressure for a few minutes. The bowels can be emptied after a while for better cleansing. If one does not wish to take enema in the lying position he can take it in the standing position.

Special Note: Enema should be taken after going to latrine. Salt can be mixed in water instead of lemon juice. You can use plain water also. Soap should not be mixed in water.

Precautions

1. Enema should be taken once in a week or in a month by a healthy person.
2. It can be taken for two to four days daily in constipation.
3. Take rest for half an hour after enema.
4. Do not take any thing after enema for an hour.

Benefits

1. Removes constipation.
2. Cleans bowels.
3. Beneficial in all diseases of stomach.

Neti

It is mainly of two types :

(*i*) Jala Neti (*ii*) Sutra Neti.

Jala Neti

For doing this, squat on your feet. Take tepid salted water in a medium sized pot with along spout, made especially for this purpose.

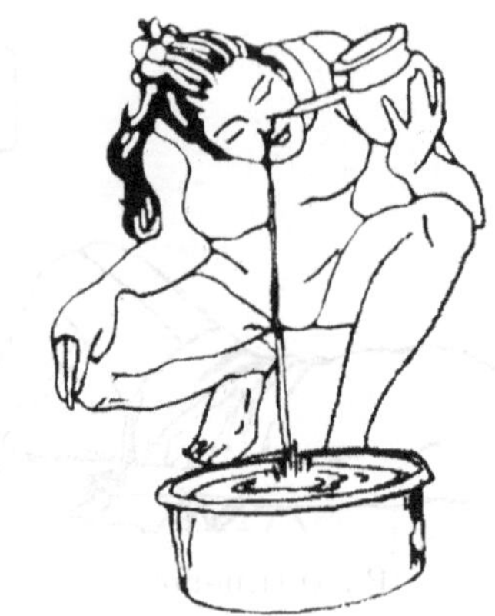

Jala Neti

Now fill the pot with tepid salted water and hold it in your right hand to the level of your nose. Then tilt your head slightly to the left so as to have the slanting position of the left nostril. Insert the nozzle of the spout into the right nostril and allow the water to flow down slowly. The water should continue falling down from other nostril in a continuous thin stream. Now repeat the process from the other side. Breath through the mouth only till the kriya is complete. After Jal Neti, stand erect with your feet together. Keep the hands behind your back clasped and blow out vigorously whatever trace of water that has remained in your nostrils.

Precautions: If sometimes one feels intolerable pain in the back of ear or above nostrils, he should practise the Kriya of Kapalbahti at once. It will cure the pain.

Water can come out of eyes in beginning of Neti. These can be warmed. Do not fear.

Benefits

- It cures sinusitis and clears sinuses.
- It cures diseases of nose, eyes, throat and prevents the occurrence of diseases.
- It purifies mind.
- It improves memory.
- It cures coryza and removes old accumulated phlegm.

Sutra Neti or Rubber Neti

Sutra Neti is performed with a 12 inches long piece of waxed cord. It is partly twisted and it makes the nasal insertion possible.

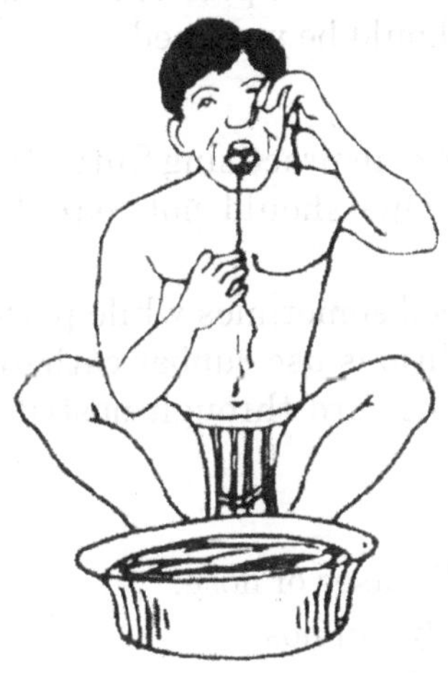

Sutra Neti

Squat on your feet. Take tepid salted water and soak the Neti well in it. Now take the waxed and twisted end of the cord and make it to curve. Bend your head slightly forward and insert the end of the cord into the nostril through which you have been breathing at that time. Push the cord gradually through the nose, down the throat. Now open your mouth wide, put your index and middle fingers in and with their tips catch the inside end of the cord and draw it out. Hold both the ends in you hand separately and pull the cord very gently up and down three to four times. Then take it out, wash it and then repeat the cycle with the other nostril.

After completion of the kriya, wash the cord with soap well and leave it to dry in some clean and safe place so that the flies, etc. do not pollute it.

Special Note

- When the cord reaches throat through nostrils, it becomes greasy by mucous. Therefore, both the ends of the cord should be caught firmly.

- Sutra Neti or Rubber Neti should be practised after learning Jal Neti. After this one can practise Neti with milk, oil or ghee.
- It is more beneficial to perform this Sutra Neti by cotton cord but it should be wrapped.

Precautions

- One can sneeze in practising Sutra Neti. Water can come out of eyes. One should not fear. Practise makes one perfect.
- Nose can bleed sometimes while performing Sutra Neti. In such conditions use rubber catheter instead of cotton cord. Move the cord through nostrils and throat slowly and gently.

Benefits

- It cures all diseases of nose.
- It reduces polyp in nose.
- It cures sinusitis.
- It cures coryza.
- It improves eyesight.
- It improves memory.
- It purifies mind.

Nasapan

Drinking water through nostrils is called nasapan. One should clean the nostrils before drinking water through them.

Milk Neti

Milk is used in place of water. Milk should be without malai cream.

Benefits: Nasapan prevents cold and coryza. It improves eyesight.

Oil Neti

Mustard oil should be made warm in a spoon. When it is lukewarm and tolerable to the skin, lie down on a bed and drip five or seven drops of oil through some dropper in both the nostrils and try to draw them in. You will feel that the oil going in. You can use clean cotton instead of Dropper. Coconut or almond oil can be used in place of mustard oil. Pure ghee can also be used. Three or four drops of ghee or Badam Rogan are sufficient for the nostrils.

Oil Neti or Neti of ghee should be done before going to bed at night.

Benefits: It lubricates noses and cleanses it. It prevents from cold and coryza.

Tratak

It is an amazing exercise to improve your power of concentration and eyesight.

It can be practised with a candle or with a black dot on a piece of paper fixed on the wall. Start this practice in a closed room, as there will be less objects to disturb your concentration.

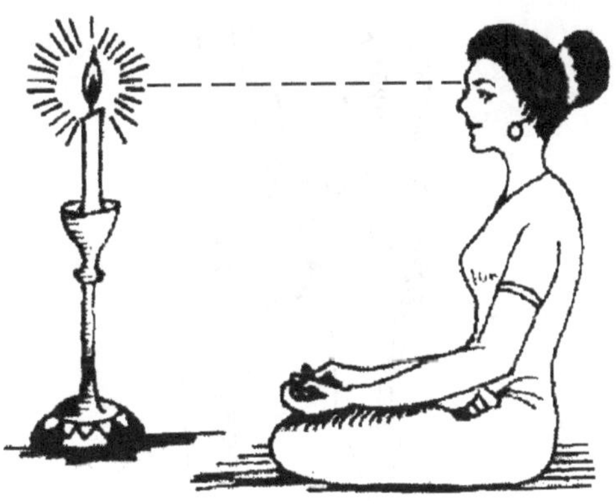

Tratak

Sit on floor in any comfortable of Padmasana pose. Keep your back and spinal cord erect. Have a few deep breaths. Make your breath steady, even and rhythmic. Keep the object of your gaze at your eye level at a distance of three to four feet. Keep the eyes meditatively wide out of your eyes. Close the eyes to let tears trickle down.

Now mentally visualize that object when the mental image visualizes, open your eyes and start gazing afresh. Do not strain your nerves and get relaxed. Let not your mind wander. Try to bring your mind back to the object but without straining yourself much as that would sap your energy and you will be tired soon.

After practising with the point on the walls or on a steady flame, try to do it concentrating on the tip of your nose on the point between the eyebrows.

Benefits

1. Tratak improves eyesight and removes the diseases of eyes.
2. It helps in concentrating your mind.
3. It purifies your mind.

Nauli Kriya

It is the best exercise for preserving and promoting the health of abdominal viscera.

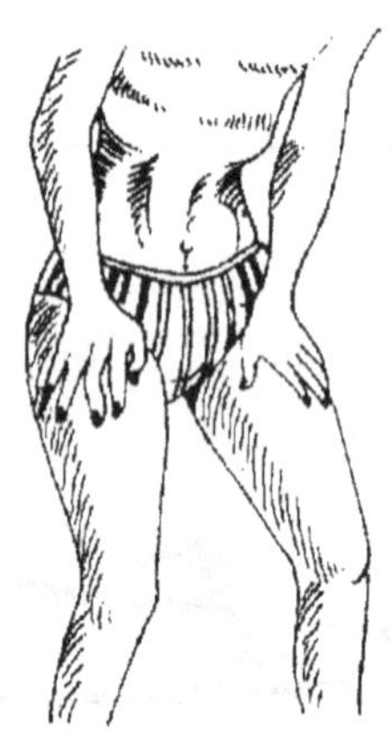

Nauli Kriya

- Nauli is equal to Uddiyana Bandh.
- Nauli should be practised daily in the morning on empty stomach and evacuated bowels.
- Stand with legs one foot apart. Bend the legs a little and stoop forward. Rest the palms on thighs just above your knees, with fingers spread. Press the thighs well with your palms and the chest with your chin at the notch between the collar bones.

- Inhale deeply and exhale vigorously so as to force out all the air from the lungs.
- Suspend the breath and pull the abdominal region back towards the spine so that a hollow is formed.
- Push the abdominal recti forward so that a vertical ridge down the centre is formed. Remain in this position for a few seconds and then relax the gap and inhale smoothly.
- Breath deeply three to four times and then repeat the cycle. Repeat it five to seven times.

Spccial Note

1. Nauli kriya is not easy. Obese persons feel difficulty in its practise. It is essential to practice Uddiyana Bandh and Agnisar to perform Nauli.
2. Nauli kriya should be performed on empty stomach after cleaning bowels and before taking food.
3. One should wear only underwear while practising Nauli. Women can wear bra/ brassiere also.

Precautions

1. Nauli should be practised on empty stomach.
2. It should not be practised unless there is some expert to demonstrate and then to guide and supervise the whole process.
3. It should not be practised before the age of 12 or 13 years.
4. The ulcer patient and the weak person should perform Nauli on the advice of Yoga therapist.
5. The patients suffering from swelling of intestines, dysentery, hernia and high blood pressure should not practice Nauli.

Benefits: The benefits of Nauli are many. It strengthens the abdominal muscles and liver. Women who suffer from a menstrual problem get immediate relief. It increases gastric fire and helps eliminating the toxic elements from the digestive system. It also helps in ovarian insufficiency. Nauli quickly cures constipation, dyspepsia, flatulence etc.

Kapalbhati

Kapal means skull. Bhati means shine or lustre. Thus, this term means "skull shining". Kapalbhati is a Pranayama also besides one of the six cleaning exercises. Actually this kriya or cleansing process is a milder form of Bhastrika, another vigorously breathing exercise.

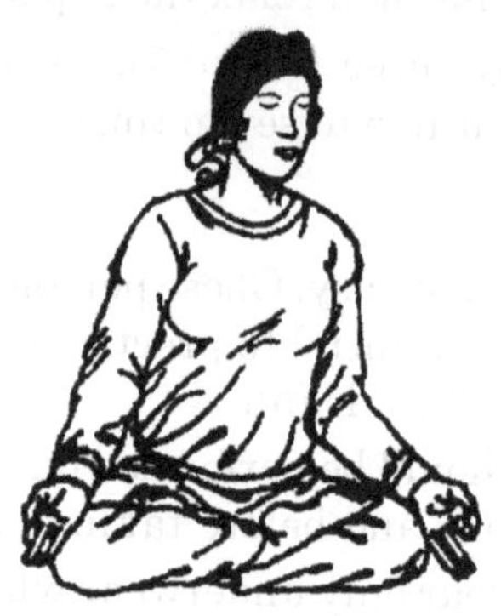

Kapalbhati

Sit on a blanket or a dari in Padmasana, Sidhasana or Sukhasana. Keep back, spinal cord and neck erect. Keep both the hands on knees. Shut your eyes. Sit peacefully. Exhale vigorously. Do not inhale. At start begin slowly after four to five exhales exhale vigorously and quickly. Be careful in exhaling; you will inhale between exhales.

One should not pause during the practice of Kapabhati. Hold the breath after exhaling (Kumbhak). During Kumbhak practice Jallandhar Bandh, Uddiyana Bandh, Mool Bandh and Mahabandh. Hold this position for a while. Release all Bandhs and inhale slowly. This completes one round of Kapalbhati. Start with two rounds. You can practice unto five rounds gradually. Start with ten or twelve exhales. Gradually you can increase their number 50 to 120.

Special Note

1. The stomach should go inside at once after exhaling.
2. The difference between Kapalbhati and Bhasrika

Pranayam is that both inhale and exhale are done vigorously. One should learn it from an expert in Yogic Kriya.

Precautions: Persons with high BP problems or pus in the ear should refrain from doing this exercise.

Benefits: This Kapalbhati is very good invigorating exercise which cleanses the entire respiratory system by forcefully rushing exhalation.

It removes concentration and mental retention. The movement of the diaphragm stimulates the stomach, heart, liver and spleen. This exercise is very good for eyes.

Agnisar

The practice of Agnisar kindles energy in stomach and body perspires.

Sit on a blanket or dari in Vajrasana. Keep a little distance between the knees. Put firmly both the hands on the knees. Inhale vigorously and while exhaling shrink your stomach as much as you can. Now suspend your breath. It is called Bahya Kumbhak.

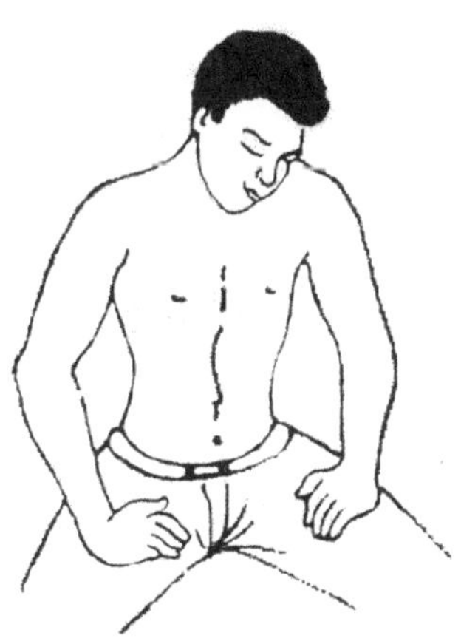

Agnisar

Holding the position of Bahya Kumbhak, i.e. Keeping the breath suspended and pulling the entire abdominal region back towards your spine. Now blow your stomach out and shrink in. In one Kumbhak you can blow and shrink your stomach 8-20 times.

This kriya is called Agnisar. One can practice this kriya in a standing posture.

Benefits

1. Cures obesity.
2. Cures disorders of abdominal region.
3. It improves lack of appetite.

❑

35
BANDHA (LOCKS)

This is a very very powerful and important practice of Yoga. It is very helpful in gaining perfect control over all the parts of the body and nerves. Bandha (lock) means to tie up or to make something stiff or to keep under control. It massages the internal organs. Although it is a physical practice that makes the functioning of body balanced and helps in attaining to better health, yet, at the same time, it also controls the thoughts and vibrations from the soul and has a subtle effect on the chakras. Thus, lock leads to spiritual progress and activation of the dormant powers in the body. In other words, Lock helps in removing the obstruction in the susumna channel and in promoting free flow of pranic energy through it. This leads to activation of several glands and helps one to have the highest experience of Yoga.

It is for this final accomplishment of liberation that asanas, pranayama, mudras and bandhas are practised. Hence, through perfect harmony between the Yogic processes, the spiritual energies are activated and spiritual powers are attained and one reaches one's final goal.

Bandha Locks

Jalandhara Bandha

(Water Gate Lock or Chin Lock)

Sit in padmasana or siddhasana or perform this practice while standing. Place the hands on the knees. Relax the entire body and close the eyes. Breathe in, deeply and, then, hold the breath in.

Bend the head forward and press the chin into the chest. Straighten the hands and pressing the knees sit still or be standing still. Position the shoulders a bit forward with both of them raised a bit. Keep the entire body, stiff and still. This is the position of Jalandhara bandha. Hold the breath in, i.e., internal retention and try to remain in this position for as long as you can, comfortably. Then, relax the shoulders and hands and raise the head. Breathe out, slowly. Rest, for some time and, then, repeat.

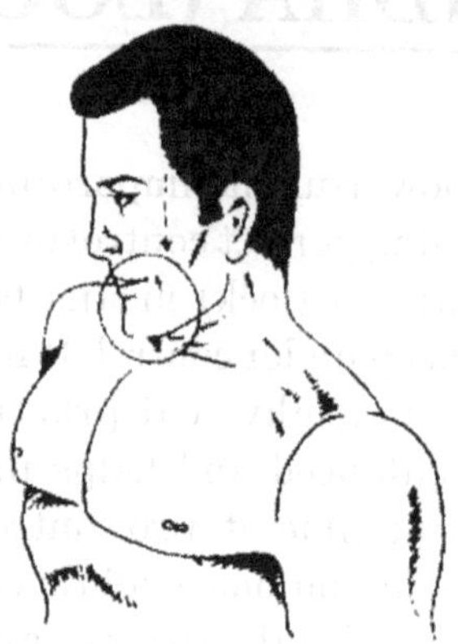

Bandha Locks

One can also perform the Bandha in another way. Breathe in deeply, then, without holding in the breath, breathe out, completely. Then, perform the bandha holding the breath out, i.e., external retention. Concentrate on the vishuddhi chakra.

Precautions: Those suffering from high blood pressure, heart problems, mental stress and migraine should practice under the guidance of a Yoga expert.

Benefits: This practice affects the nerves of the neck, the arteries that carry blood to the head, the thyroid and parathyroid glands, etc. Thus, the shape and development of the body and the sexual performance get regulated. It also helps in getting rid from mental tension, worries, anger and mental disorders. It also helps control disorders related to high and low blood pressure.

Mula Bandha (Root Lock or the Anal Lock)

Sit in any meditative pose with the knees touching the floor. For this, siddhasana is best. In this lock, the muladhara region is contracted. Thus, mula bandha, i.e., the anal lock is performed, automatically. Close the eyes and place the palms on the knees. Relax the entire body. Breathe in deeply and hold the breath in, i.e., internal tension. Then, perform Jalandhara bandha. Contract and relax the sphincter muscles and try to pull them, inwards. This is the final position. Try to hold the breath in for as long as you can and keep contracting and relaxing the sphincter muscles. Finally, relax the muscles and relax the Lock. Then, slowly breathe out. Concentrate on the midadhara chakra.

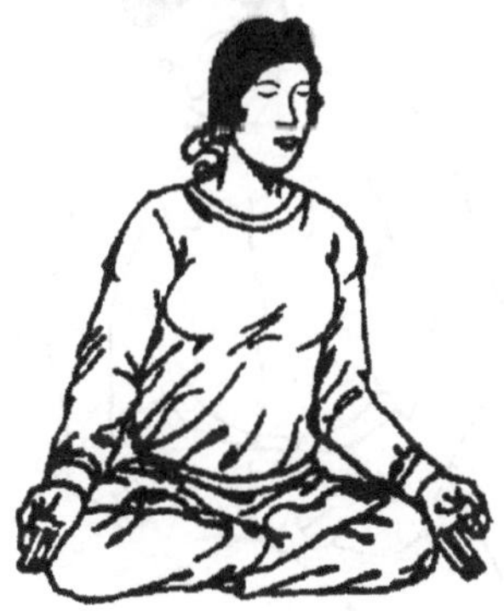

Mula Bandha

One can also do this practice after exhaling, completely and holding the breath out, i.e., external retention. Those who wish to remain in the final position for a long time can do so by breathing, normally.

Benefits: In this practice, the apana vayu mixes with prana vayu, i.e., the excretory air merges into the life force called as vital air and this results in generation of a great amount of energy that helps in activation,of kundalin more easily. This practice is helpful in maintenance of celibacy and activation of divine energy within. It is also very beneficial for those suffering from piles, indigestion and other stomach ailments. It tones up and strengthens the sphincter muscles, the nerves of the waist region and the intestines. It prepares the mind for spiritual practices.

Uddiyana Bandha (Abdominal Lock)

Sit in a meditative pose in which the knees touch the floor. Padmasana and Sidhasana are best. Place the palms on the knees. Breathe out, completely and holding the breath out, i.e., external retention perform Jalandhara bandha. Now, pull the stomach inwards and upwards as much as you can, i.e., total contraction of abdomen. Remain in the final position comfortably. Type of worshipping can also be of three types–Vedic, smarta and laukika.

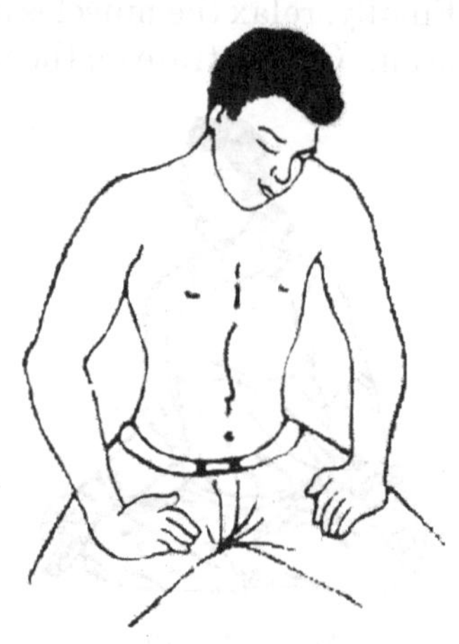

Uddiyana Bandha

For Vedic worship, one has to, first, learn the proper pronunciation of the Vedic mantras and also know about the (the seer of the mantra), chanda (the metre of the mantra), devata (deity), brija (the code of the mantra), gakti (the trigger), Maka (lock and viniyoga (the offering) related to a particular mantra, the syllable. One has to daily have a bath before starting the practice. One has to wear fresh clothes, sit on a particular worship-mat with a pure heart and meditate on the divine form of the deity, after having performed rsyadi nyasa (establishing the etc., in our body in different specific organs who created that particular practice), (to establish the diety, etc., in the different parts of our body) and karanyasa (to establish the deity, etc., in the different fingers of our hand). These are very essential for the purification of all the parts of our body, before using a particular practice for prayer, without which the deity cannot be pleased. If there is a special verse for meditation, then, one should contemplate on the divine form of the deity in one's heart and devote oneself on his feet. Thereafter, one should chant the Vedic mantra 2, 3, 5, 11, 21, 51, 108 or, more times, with full concentration. In the end, one should offer one's chanting into the feet of the deity to appease.

❑

36
QUICK CUR BY MUDRAS

There are several mudras but I have described here only those which are of much benefit.

Gyan Mudra

In Yoga Shastra this Mudra signified as the 'Gyan Mudra' Here top of index finger is touched with top portion of the thumb, and our saints/yogis have immensely practised on this mudra.

Lord Buddha and Lord Mahavira have been shown in this mudra. In the battle field of Kurukshetra Lord Krishna explained the intricacies of *Geeta* to Arjun in the same Mudra hence its utmost importance.

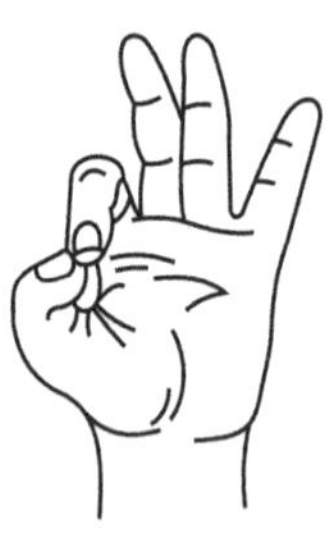

Gyan Mudra

Thumb signifies Fire element and the index finger represents/signifies Air element. When both the elements conjoin, Gyan Mudra comes into existence and air element gets established and balanced. By continuous practice of this Mudra, malfunction of symptoms-blood vessels of the brain can be set in order, without aid of any medicine. In addition, irregular and disturbed sleep, weak memory, anger, insanity can be easily dispelled. It also enhances receptive capability whereby a person is able to acquire and sore knowledge, all around him, in his brain. Persons, whose mental activity has been weakened, should regularly practise this mudra. This mudra is an attribute of Yogic meditation or trance (Samadhi), and is practised to concentrate. Its regular practice fortifies and strengthens nerves.

Vairagya Mudra

Sit in Padmasana, Siddhasana or in any comfortable asana, whichever suits you best. Place both the hands, as was done in Gyan Mudra, on your knees in an upward position, and sit quietly and peacefully. This mudra is formed by touching frontal portion of the thumb with index finger's frontal portion. Swami Dayanad spent major part of his time by sitting in this posture. Most of his devotees are seen sitting in this posture while they have to chant mantra'. After 'Gyan' Vairagya' (Renunciation) is the next step. Hence Vairagaya and Gyan mudras are practised in unison. This mudra inculcates and develops spirituality and imparts self-knowledge. The devotee becomes mentally and physically healthy, and his spiritual knowledge is also added.

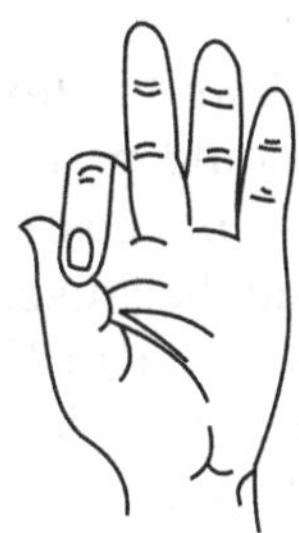

Vairagya Mudra

Abhaya Mudra

The practitioner should form Gyan Mudra with both of his hands, and place his hands along side the shoulders as shown in the above picture. As the name of this mudra indicates, it inculcates courage and solid determination in a person. 'Gyan' is followed by 'Vairagya' and self-confidence is the natural outcome of complete knowledge. If practised regularly, it will bring a permanent benefit to a devotee's mind, brain and heart; and he will be relieved permanently from the mental tension and agony. The bigger achievement through this mudra being that a person will not get horrified by fear or any sort of calamity. In ancient times the sages and ascetics used to practise Sadhana in the forests. This mudra kept them free from the fear of fierce animals and other problems and, thus, they used to feel courageous and bold.

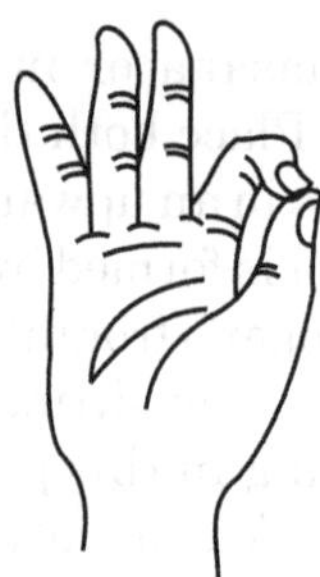

Abhaya Mudra

Dhyana Mudra

To make a pose for Dhyana Mudra a person should place his hands in the same position as are placed in Gyan Mudra that is frontal portion of his thumb and index finger should touch with each other and then he should place the same upon his laps, while sitting in any comfortable posture. This mudra also helps in concentration of the mind, because, as the mudras explained earlier, base of this mudra is also the Gyan Mudra. Dhyana Mudra, if practised regularly for a longer span of time, imparts a unique and divine bliss. It is also very useful for mental agony and agitation. In addition, it also keeps blood pressure under control.

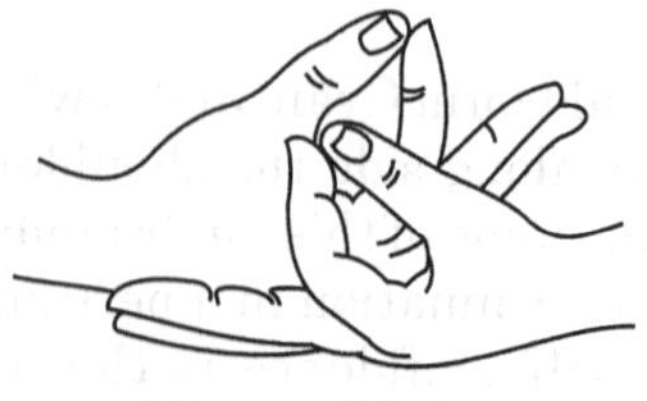

Dhyana Mudra

Vaayu Mudra

Turn the index finger and touch it with the base (root) of the thumb, exerting very light pressure. Index finger controls air element (one of the five elements) and any imbalance in air element can emerge in the form of wind related diseases. Vaayu Mudra effectively treats many wind related incurable diseases like gout, polio paralysis, trembling or Parkinson's diseases and acts as a medicine.

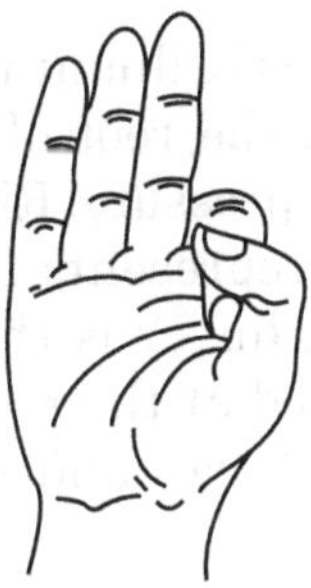

Vaayu Mudra

Shoonya Mudra

If the middle finger's tip is touched at the root (base of the thumb as shown in the picture) it forms Shoonya mudra.

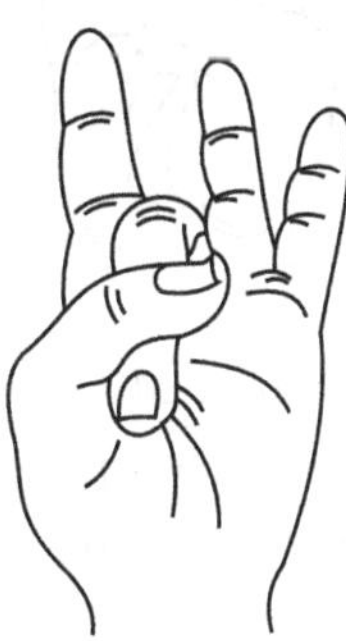

Shoonya Mudra

Shoonya represents sky (or Vacuum) element, and is synonym of the sky. Sky element is present in even in a minute object of this universe, apart from it the same element is present in every part of our body. When this element gets disbalanced, many diseases surface. Vaccum element is directly related to sound, hence due to its disbalance, many ear related diseases ensue. When there is a pain in the ear, it can be subsided quickly if this mudra is practised at the inception stage of pain and thus, many ear related problems like discharges from the ear, chronic ear ache, deafness and hard of hearing can be cured effectively, if this mudra is practised for 45 minutes daily.

Surya Mudra

As the name indicates, it is brilliant mudra. Join or touch your ring finger (Anamika) at the root of thumb (as shown in the picture) maintaining light pressure. Ring finger represents earth element, and the thumb represents fire element. According to Saamudrik Shastra, ring finger is the seat of the sun. Hence, when ring finger is pressed at the root of the thumb, plenty of energy is generated which can and should be compared with solar energy.

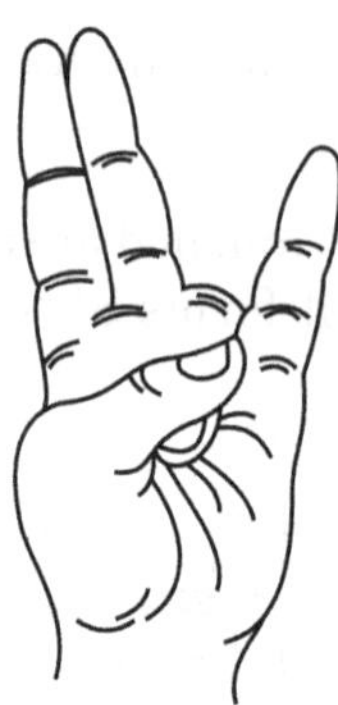

Surya Mudra

Surya Mudra is particularly effective in curing any type of headache or sense of heaviness in the brain. It also resolves problem of obesity.

Varun Mudra

Varun Mudra is formed by joining the little finger's top with the top of the thumb. The little finger represents water element. By continuous practice of this mudra, all the diseases that are caused by lassitude of water element, can be treated. It also imparts glow and smoothness to the face.

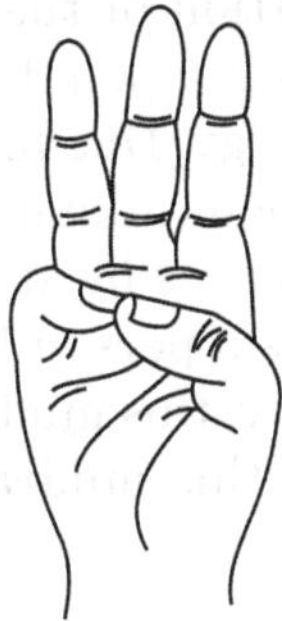

Varun Mudra

It also removes roughness from the face, apart from removing facial wrinkles and purifying the blood, it also restores elegance and cleanliness to the face.

Prithvi Mudra

Prithvi Mudra is formed by touching the frontal position of the thumb with the frontal portion of the ring finger. By practising this mudra tones down earth element is compensated and enhanced. It also enhances other elements in the body due to which body remains healthy and proper balance among all the elements remain well maintained. If body weight is less than the height of the body, this mudra restores proper proportion and balance between both the facets. Its practice also imparts lustre, glow and brightness to the face, and also inclines and motivates the mind towards spirituality. It also installs qualities of mercy, compassion and love, in addition to tolerance and patience.

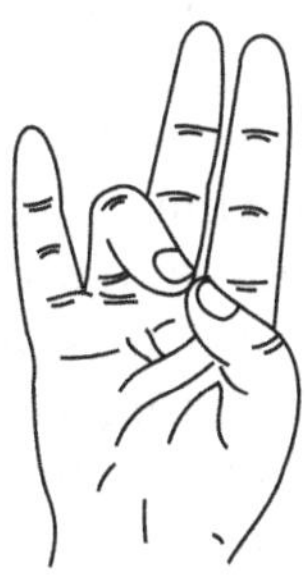

Prithvi Mudra

Prana Mudra

Prana Mudra is formed by joining the front portion of little and ring finger with front portion of the thumb. This mudra acts like an electric stick, because, when this switch, is pressed, whole body gets infused with energy. Due to lack of Pranic energy, our body is embroiled with various ailments. One can always remain healthy and free from diseases by storing pranic energy in the body and this mudra helps a person fully to achieve him object of staying healthy. In reality, this mudra actually imparts 'Pran'. By continuous practice of this mudra, all eye-related diseases can be dispelled.

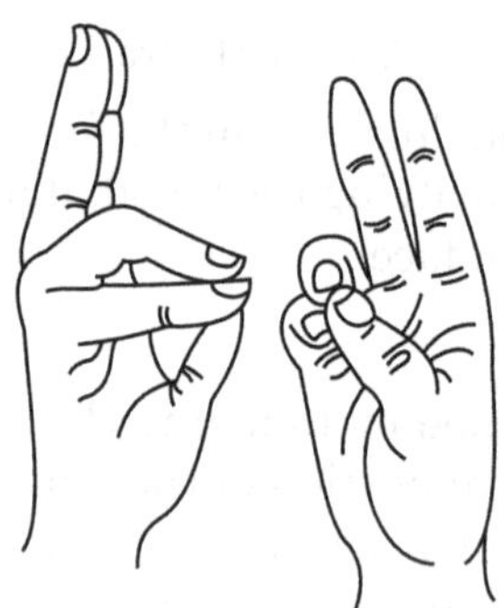

Prana Mudra

Apaan Mudra

Deficiency of inadequacy of Pran Vaayu is a causative factor for onset of many diseases. Impure and toxic matters can not be expelled from the body, if this element is found wanting, as a result of which impurities and diseases overpower human body. Hence our body can stay clear from such diseases and impurities if our body continues to utilise Apaan Vaayu thus keeping balance within all the elements. Its use is like baking the body in fire so that blood is purified and body and mind are also purified of harmful substances. If any patient is suffering from urinary obstruction, due to any reason, he will pass urine within 15-20 minutes after practising this mudra. But, patients suffering from prostate gland and stone problems will not benefit from this Mudra. To restore the urinary flow, this mudra must be performed with both the hands.

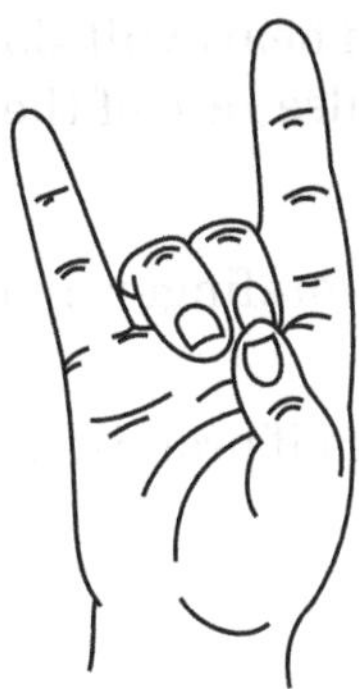

Apaan Mudra

If the pregnant ladies practise this mudra in the 8th month of pregnancy for 45 minutes daily, they will have an easy delivery and delivery will so take place at the expected time. If any pregnant lady finds it difficult to expel the baby or if delivery is getting delayed, she also can have an easy and natural delivery, provided she regularly practises this mudra.

If a person has suffered a heart attack, he should form this mudra with his left hand and also firmly compresses his right hand's thumb, middle and ring fingers himself or asks some another person to do the job for him, he will have an instant relief. This experiment has been used on many patients of heart attack and at all the occasions we were successful.

If a person has vomiting and loose motions (diarrhoea), he must not practise this mudra as he is most likely to be harmed.

Apan Mudra

Method: Bend the forefinger to touch the base of the thum and join the tips of middle finger and ring finger with the thip of thumb.

Benefits: This mudra has proved to be the most wonderful treatment for coronary ailments. In emergency cases (like heart attack), this mudra shows its immediate effect on the heart patients like the sorbitrate tablet and patient gets miraculous relief in the form of first aid. That is why it is also called

'Mirtsanjivani Mudra'. If this mudra is practised regularly for a short period of time, then heart will slowly become quite strong. It also normalizes the pulse rate of the person.

Vyan Mudra

Method: Join the tip of forefinger and middle finger to the tip of thumb.

Benefits: This mudra if practised continuously reduces the High Blood Pressure.

❑

37
SURYA NAMASKAR: 12 SIMPLE STEPS

Sun is supposed to be the best source of energy. The Asana by which Sun is worshipped is called 'Surya namaskar'. This consists of 12 steps and with every step, Sun is worshipped by a specific Mantra.

This asana is supposed to be complete in itself. Any body, of any sex, at any age, this can be performed. This should be done smoothly and slowly. No other asana should be performed before or after Surya Namaskar. Neither jogging nor brisk walking is required before or after Surya Namaskar. This asana should be performed by keeping face towards Sun in early morning.

Caution: Patients/Persons suffering from heart problems, having B.P. alterations or during fever, this asana should not be performed.

First Step: Stand on a blanket or mat keeping your face in front of the Sun. Join the knees, heels and feet of both legs. Keep your back, spinal cord and head in a straight position. Join both the hands and bend the elbow in a position of Namaskar. This is first step. Now repeat silently–'OM Mitroya Namah'. (Friend Sun, I salute you).

Second Step: Raise your both arms by inhaling. Stop breathing. Keeping air inside your lungs. Bend your back, neck, head and arms backwards. Legs should not bend and keep your body in this position for some seconds. This is second step. Repeat–(OM Ravya Namah) in your mind. (May Sun! you are capable of keeping this world mobile so I salute you).

Third Step: Now release your holded breath and bend yourself forward. Touch your both palms to earth and your forehead should touch the knees. There should be no bend in knees. This is third step. repeat in your mind–'OM Suryay Namah' (Sun, you are capable of providing life to this world, so I salute you).

Fourth Step: The palms should be touched to earth and start inhaling. Raise your left leg backwards. Bend your right knee and keep it on Sole. Keep your chest ahead. Bend your neck backwards. Look forwards sky. This is fourth step. Recall Sun in your mind with the Mantra–'OM Bhanve Namah' (Hey! source of light, I salute you).

Fifth Step: Straight your both arms, keeping your palms on the earth. Start taking breath and raise your right leg too backwards. Now keep both the legs parallel. But there should be no gap in between heela and knees of both legs. The whole weight of the body should be on palms and soles. Now repeat in mind–'OM Khagaya Namah' (Hey! Sun you are able for motion in sky, I salute you).

Sixth Step: Hold the breath in lungs and keeping your palms and soles on earth, bend your elbows and touch your chest and knees to earth. This is called 'Ashtaang Pranaam'. In this position light organs of the body touch the earth i.e. two soles, two hands, chest, forehead and two knees; so why it is called 'Ashtaang Pranaam'. This is the sixth step. Now remember Sun by repeating in your mind–'OM Pushney Namah'–(Hey! Sun, you are providing food to world, I salute you).

Seventh Step: Keep your palms on the earth and straight your arms, keeping breath. Raise your upper portion of the body upto naval pit. Keep ahead your chest and bend your neck backwards. Look forwards sky. Raise your legs backwards, keeping your soles towards sky. This is step seven. Now repeat–'OM Hiranya Garbhaya Namah'–(As you are a light source, I salute you).

Eighth Step: Keep your palms on the earth. Exhale the breath and raise both the legs towards hands. Raise the hips straight. Keep soles, feet and palms in touch of earth. Keep your head in between of the arms. Raise your back. There should be no gap in between both legs. Keep your stomach inside & hold the breath outside. Now remember Sun by repeating in mind– 'Om Marichaye Namah'–(Sun, you are all in all, so I salute you).

Ninth Step: Continue the retention of breath. Place hands and feet firmly on the ground. Lift your bottoms. Press your chin to the chest. Stomach should be drawn in.

Tenth Step: While sitting on the ground, put the left foot forward and right foot backwards stretchingly. Try to touch your front foot with your fingers of hands. The throat should be between the two arms and erect. Stomach should be drawn in. Bring the right foot forward and draw the left foot backwards stretchingly. Try to touch the front foot with fingers of both hands. This improves blood circulation, strengthens the feet and makes the spinal cord elastic.

Eleventh Step: Drawing the stomach in join both legs. Touch the knees with your nose. Exhale with nose. This strengthens fingers, hands, chest and stomach.

Twelfth Step: Inhale with nose. Stand erect and join feet and knees. Keep the hands folded and touching firmly your chest.

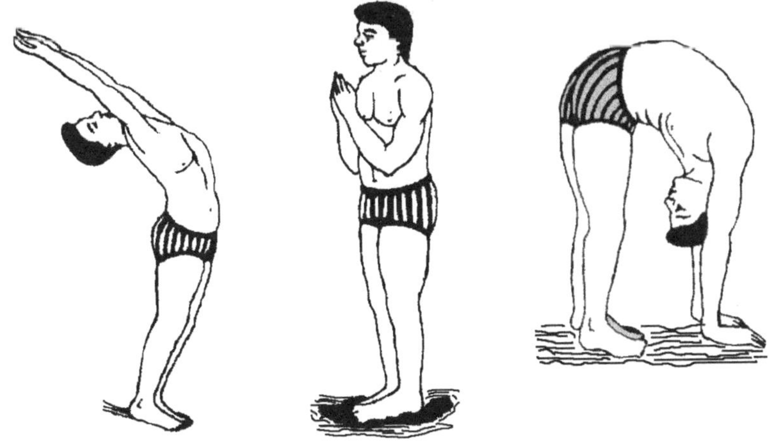

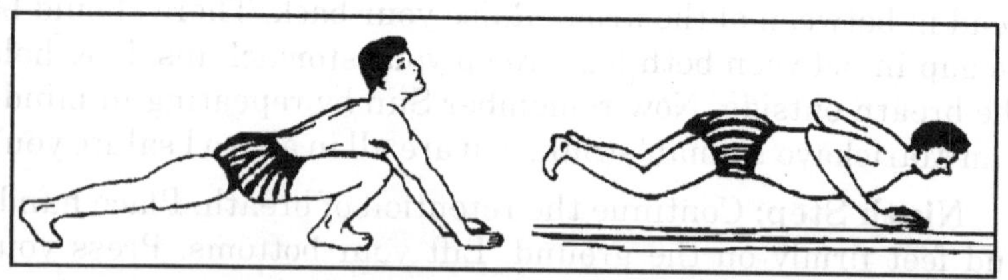

Advantages of Surya Namaskar

- By practising Surya Namaskar in winter, you will be free from cold, cough and coryza.
- Eye sight is improved.
- Shoulders are strengthened and abdominal diseases are cured.
- The mind becomes tension free and mind power is increased.
- The spinal cord becomes elastic and muscles are strengthened surrounding spinal cord.
- Blood circulation of whole body is accelerated and diseases of respiratory system are annihilated.
- Ligaments are strengthened.
- Body becomes vigorous and glowing.

❑

38
PRANA VIDYA (SCIENCE OF VITAL ENERGY)

We have already described prana, Science of Pranayama. In brief, the divine life-force that enters the body along with the air we breathe in, is prana. Several types of pranayama have been described for achieving control over prana through the control of breathing. This is done for spiritual and physical gains. The highest science relating to prana is called prana-vidya. By practising the process being revealed, here, one can gain the capability of using, prana for the physical and spiritual good of oneself and others, too.

One can, do this practice while sitting, lying on the back or on the stomach or lying on the side. The only thing is that the spine should be straight. One should do this practice, when the right nostril is working, i.e., when the pingala channel is active. This practice is done in two steps. In the first step, while breathing in, imagine that pranic energy is flowing from the manipara chakra or each pore of the body towards chakra and accumulating there.

Then, slowly breathe out. In the second step, imagine that the accumulated pranic energy is being disseminated to all parts of the body through the various spiritual channels. Or imagine it is flowing to that part of the body where you have some pain, disease or any other part, where you want it to concentrate for special benefit. If you wish it to flow into the body of some person, use the thumb and the ring finger of the right hand to transfer the energy to the desired part of the body.

Procedure: Close the eyes lightly and become ready. Get into a comfortable position but with the spine straight and be still. Now harmonize the pace of the flow of prana with the pace of breathing.

Remember that the pranic energy moves in circles, anticlockwise. Imagine the pranic energy starting from the muladhara and moving up in a semi-circle from the right to reach the svadhisthana. Then, from there, it moves again in a semi-circle but from the left to the manipura chakra. In this manner, it rises up from one chakra to another until it reaches the chakra. Then, it returns to the muladhara from the reverse direction. This is the conscious flow of the pranic energy in wave form.

When you have become perfect in this practice, then, let the pranic energy rise, as you breathe in and, let it return, as you breathe out, normally. Also be aware of the whole process as the pranic energy rises and gets accumulated in a waveless form in the aftia chakra. Repeat in your mind that both your pranic energy and your conscious energy are getting accumulated in the ajna chakra.

After this, hold the breath in and perform the three bandhas and feel the kundalini power rising to the chakra along with the pranic energy. Relax the bandhas and breathe out. Then, let the body relax. Repeat the cycle again. Imagine that you are not breathing in and out just through the nostrils but through every pore of the body. Each time you breathe in, feel the pranic energy and the kundalini rising; and every time you breathe out, feel the body relaxing.

Then breathe in, deeply and slowly. Feel that the breath is spreading to each part of the body and the accumulated pranic energy in the chakra is being disseminated throughout the body. The pranic energy is not only flowing up and down through the chakras in the spine, but is reaching every cell of the body. The breathing should be in the form of ujjayi pranayama.

Further, imagine that you are breathing not through the nostrils or the body pores but through the chakra. With each inhalation, feel the entire body being filled with pranic energy and with each exhalation, feel the body relaxing. Feel this with a harmony between the breathing, the imagination, the inner vision, the feelings, the thoughts and the awareness of the body. Do not concentrate on just one. Feel that your body is blowing like a balloon, as all these processes go on. The body shall expand as you breathe in and relax as you breathe out. Also, there shall be dissemination of the pranic energy and relaxation of the body, respectively.

When you have mastered this practice, try to make the pranic energy flow wilfully through the various parts of the body. In the end, again, let the pranic energy disseminate with inhalation and let the body relax with exhalation. Thereafter, open the eyes. For the best use of such practices and quick progress in them, one needs the guidance of a capable guru. Do not try to do on your own. Otherwise there might be reverse results instead of benefits.

Kundalini Vidya
(Science of Kundalini: The Dormant Energy)

This is the highest form of dhyana and sadhana, i.e., meditation and spiritual practices. One should try to do this practice after getting initiation from a guru.

❑

39
DIET FOR THE REIKI PRACTITIONERS

A well balanced diet contains sufficient quality of protein, carbohydrates, fats, salts and minerals. It is said in Reiki that "as you eat, so you become". This is because the kind and quality of food affects the physical as well as mental conditions of the individual. In Yoga all foods have been divided into three categories: Rajasi (Royal), Tamasi (Carnal) and Satvik (Noble). The Rajasi food comprises a variety of dishes. This type of food includes fried, roasted and fatty stuff, which is not desirable for good health. A little intake of these types should be sufficient to titillate the palate. A little quantity of strongly spiced bitter or sour food (Tamasik) should also form part of diet which should mostly be made easily digestible, nourishing; and freshly prepared food which classifies the noble or Satvik food. Your food must give you the variety of all the six varieties of taste–sweet, salty, astringent, bitter, sour and biting. However, it is not only the quantity or quality of the food but your way of eating which is also very important. Whatever food you eat, masticate it thoroughly and allow the saliva to reduce the eaten morsel to a mere puop before gulpig it down. Always eat 75 to 80% of your total capacity and leave enough room for the movement of gas/liquid etc. to help the system digest the eaten food quickly. Drinking water with food should be totally forgotten. Drink water always half an hour before and half an hour after your having food. Drink enough of water between your meals but not with it.

For your help we are giving below some guidelines following which you shall remain healthy. Adherence to them will not only keep diseases and disorders at bay but enhance also the age of your healthy life.

- The food that we eat helps build the blood cells, nerves, bones and muscles in our body. It has been proved scientifically that food which is highly processed and high in protein, fat, salt and sugar leads to health problems. Nutritious food (balanced wholesome diet, moderate exercises, drinking enough water, that is 8/10 glasses (3 litres) of water, enjoying fresh air and sunshine, resting adequately every day, will ensure a healthy body and mind.
- Detoxify the system completely by fasting 2 to 4 days every three months with liquids, preferably fresh lemon water with honey 4-5 times daily and follow it up with an all fruit course for 5 to 7 days and then resort to normal diet, cautiously and gradually. Take enema on the days of fasting immediately after taking mud pack for 15/20 minutes. Also take abdominal pack at night.
- Abdoment must be kept cool and soft always. All liquid intake should be close to the body temperature as far as possible. Take mud pack, hip bath, enema and oil massage intermittently.
- Drink 1 or 2 glasses of water on rising, every morning.
- Dental health plays a vital role in curing a troubled abdomen. An unhealthy abdomen; an unhealthy abdomen is responsible for most of the diseases.
- Use honey and molasses instead of sugar. Use a lot of garlic and some ginger if they suit. Take maximum roughage/fibre.
- Avoid non-vegetarian, concentrated, stimulating, intoxicating and gas forming foods.
- Ideal time for lunch is 10.00 a.m. and for dinner 7.00 p.m. May take some fruits (one variety only) around 2.00 p.m. Take only two meals a day and satisfy 80% of your hunger or appetite. Do not eat if not hungry or in bad mood/anger or at odd hours.

- Shun smoking, tea, coffee, alcohol, Zarda, Pan-masala, soft drinks and drugs.
- Going for brisk walk and/or doing Yoga for 30 to 60 minutes daily is must.
- Wash vegetables and fruits properly under running water, scrubbing with a brush before cutting, as they contain pesticides and contaminates. If any germs are suspected then wash in water with diluted solution of potassium permanganate.
- Ensure good digestion,sound sleep,good appetite and evacuation of bladder and bowels regularly and naturally.
- Tension is very harmful, as it causes flatuence, constipation, irritability, besides liver and heart problems. Hence, change the way of living. do not work for long hours. Do Shavasana and enjoy minimum 7 sound sleeps daily.
- Always use polyunsaturated oil and reduce salt and sugar intake to the minimum possible level.
- After lunch, rest a while and after dinner, walk a mile - is a wise old recommendation. Relax in Vajrasana for 10-15 minutes afte the meal.
- Take very light but nutritious food which includes fruits, skimmed milk and yoghurt (curd).
- For healthy condition, 80 per cent of alkaline foods to 20 percent alkaline diet is needed. Alkaline food and drink purify the blood. Refined and processed foods tend to acidify and pollute the blood and the cells.
- Select your food from the following.

(a) Acid producing foods

All fresh foods, fish, pulses, white bread, polished rice, white flour, nuts, confectionery, sweets, coffee, tea, alcohol, boiled buffalo milk, fried foods, concentrated foods, hydrogenated stuff, beans, onions, peanuts, tomatoes, jam and all preservatives, pickles, unripe fruits, refined stuff, grapes and high protein foods.

(b) Alkali producing foods

All kinds of vegetables, potatoes, fresh fruits,butter milk, fresh lemon, coconuts, figs, dates, almonds, loquates, skimmed milk,yoghurt, molasses, sweet oranges, dry fruits, sprouts, whole flour/unpolished rice and honey.

Foods to be Replaced/limited

- Limit intake of cheese and red-meats that are high in saturated fat content.
- Number of calories, obtained from fat, must be kept below 30% of total daily dietary intake of calories.
- Not more than 10% of total fat calories should be obtained of from saturated fat intake.
- Avoid processed and junk foods that are overloaded with flavouring preservatives and colourings.
- Butter should be replaced with soft margarine or low fat foods that are high in polyunsaturated fats. Spread it thinly.
- To keep the blood sugar level within normal confines, consume sugar in limited quantity.
- Salt intake must be limited. Avoid eating salty foods, and also adding (extra) salt to meals. Also do not consume processed meats and crispy eatables.
- Limit use of tea, coffee, cold drinks, chocolates and sweets so as to reduce intake of caffeine. Instead you may use herbal teas with advantage but without hassles.
- Excessive intake of alcohol must be reduced.
- Do not use strong spices and condiments as they irritate stomach.

Ideal Menu and Timing

- On rising early in the morning, drink a glass or two of normal water.
- Take a glass of juice (carrot/apple with sweet lime/ orange) before going for a brisk walk around 7.00 a.m. (during summer 6.00 a.m.) May take a cup of skimmed milk after vigorous yogic exercises, if suits.

Lunch (10:00 a.m.)

Take nutritious food as you need enough energy for working whole day.	Take good Salad (consume first), cooked vegetables 2 or 3 cups, medium chapati 2-3 or rice 2 cups, 2 cups cooked pulse, 1 or 2 cups of youghurt (Dahi), steamed vegetables 1/2 or 1 cup.

Supper (Around 7:00) p.m.)

Out of total 1600 Calories consumed during the whole day, evening meal should not contain more than 350.	As per your taste and choice but light, e.g. (A) 1 or 2 cooked vegetables, with 1 chapati, and 1 calories cup of yoghurt or (B) 1 cup soup, 1 fruit and raw vegetables or (C) 2 cups of skimmed milk with 1 or 2 bananas or apples or toast or bread slices.

- If you have to go out for dinner, take just a cup of skimmed milk or soup or eat some roasted grams or some fruits/ vegetables at around 6:00 p.m. before going. If you take a late evening dinner, drink a glass of lemon juice (juice of 1 lemon in one glass of warm water) the following morning (empty stomach).

Herbs and Spices

- You may use asafoetida (Hing), cloves, corriander, garlic, ginger, saunf, turmeric, cumin (Jeera), cardamon, ajwain, pepper, and kali rai.
- Bed tea/coffee is very harmful. Avoid tea/coffee/cold drinks and fried items always.

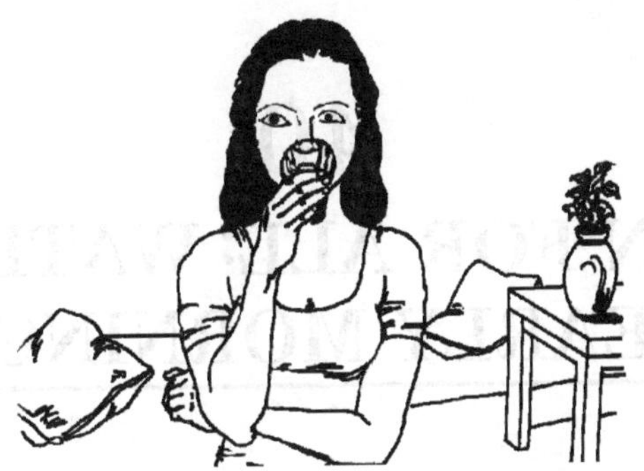

For Reiki attunement, not only one's mind but body should be pure. One should take care of purity and cleanliness of his or her eatables too.

❑

40

BOON FOR ALL: WATER IN EARLY MORNING

Water is panacea for chronic and incurable diseases. Rise early from bed. Do not wash your face and mouth as you do normally. Sit comfortably and drink four large glasses of water. Do not take any thing for 45 minutes. You can wash your face and brush your mouth after drinking water.

Always drink water after an hour of breakfast and meals. Regular intake of water in early morning gives relief in following diseases:

1. Diabetes
2. Acne, Boils
3. Headache
4. Blood pressure
5. Old age and wrinkles
6. Arthritis
7. Paralysis problem of ladies
8. Anaemia
9. Heart diseases, Faintness
10. Cold, Cough, Asthma, Bronchitis
11. Obesity
12. Meningitis
13. Disorders of liver
14. Tuberculosis
15. Disorders of the eye

16. Irregular menstruation
17. Urinary problems, Stones, etc.
18. Hyperacidity
19. Gastric trouble and diseases concerned with back, Spine
20. Cancer of ovary
21. Swelling, Fever
22. Digestive disorders
23. Piles
24. Diseases caused by Vata, Pitta, Cough.
25. Mental weakness, etc.

If sick persons or soft natured persons with a delicate physique are unable to take four glasses of water at a stretch, they should start from one or two glasses and then gradually they should start taking four glasses. Take four glasses of water regularly. Experiments have proved that different diseases can be cured within the time given below by its regular use:

Hypertension	–	Within one month
Gastric trouble	–	Within ten days
Cancer	–	Within six months
Constipation	–	Within ten days
Diabetes	–	Within one month
TB	–	Within three months
Leucorrhoea	–	Within one month
Paralysis	–	Within three months

Other diseases described above may be cured within four to six months according to their nature. Drinking four glasses of water does not have any ill-effects on health. Only urge to pass urine will be great and you will pass urine in large quantities frequently. Passing of stool will be easy and complete. It will facilitate the expulsion of the accumulated waste matter very effectively and leave you fresh. Besides hydrotherapy certain other measures or house hold remedies are also advised for such disorders.

Some Important Facts

1. Never drink water before passing urine or just after passing urine.
2. Passing urine after meals prevents formation of stones.
3. Stand on forefoot and then pass urine. This posture prevents formation of stones.
4. Water contained in copper vessel is hundred times more useful.
5. Take juice of one lemon in a glass of warm water before going to bed. It gives relief in Coryza.
6. Take juice of one lemon and tea spoon of honey in warm water in morning. It helps in curing obesity and improves complexion.
7. In early morning, chew five leaves of Neem (Azadiracta indica) and Holy Tulsi (Ocimum basilium) and drink a glass of water after chewing these leaves. This can prevent you from carcinoma (Cancer) and plague too.
8. Take a little rice (raw–one or two tea spoons) with a glass of water to cure liver disorders.
9. The water kept in a Shankh for a whole night is remedy for Stammering speech. Continue this for four to six months.

Role of Water on Stomach

There is secretion of stomachic juice in stomach to digest food. The more genuine the stomachic juice, the better digestion of food.

If someone takes liquid whether it is water, wine or beer, the stomachic juice will not remain genuine. It would be adulterated by the intake of water, wine or beer and would not be effective in digestion of food.

Similarly, if some person takes water six or eight times while taking his meal, it would liquidate stomachic juice so much that it would not be able to act as digestive juice.

Do not take water at all during meals. If you have to take it, take very small quantity of it, so that genuine stomachic juice may be absorbed in all eaten food.

If you feel thirsty after one hour or more of taking food, please take water in limited quantity. Body especially stomach needs water at interval from time to time to liquidate its juice, to increase its quantity and to absorb the solid material (food). The body itself informs whenever it needs it. Sometimes, the desire to take water is slow and someti~es it is very fast. One should be particular about intake whether it is from healthy or sick stomach. One should take it as much as it is sufficient and good for health.

It should be taken at equal intervals of time especially when one is suffering from fever. One should not take a glass of water at a stretch but each five or ten minutes in less quantity. Intake of water at a stretch by a patient of fever, will not quench his thirst, rather it would increase other symptoms of illness.

Water taken in less quantity is at once accepted and absorbed by stomach. Repetition of its intake at each half-an-hour produces juice in more quantity and removes whole dullness and constipation by flowing in body and intestines. It cools them also.

One can use luke-warm water or cold water according to its taste.

Use of Water

1. Saline water is necessary in dehydration caused by cholera, fever, diabetes, diarrhoea, etc.
2. It is useful to take water with salt, sugar, lemon and honey. Patients of kidney diseases should use water with salt in supervision of some naturopath.
3. Some of vegetables, water of pulse, sharbat of lemon and juice etc. contain water. They give us minerals and salts along with water.

❑

41
LIFESTYLE TIPS FOR REIKI PRACTITIONERS

While you are practising Reiki, you should also ensure that your lifestyle is such which keeps your energy body clean, positive and strong. This will be very favourable to your Reiki healing practices.

1. Stop or minimize caffeine drinks (e.g. coffee, tea, soft drinks, chocolate etc.). They create imbalance in the nervous and endocrine system and hence in the energy body.
2. Stop alcohol intake.
3. Minimize taking sweets white sugar products.
4. Stop or minimize smoking.
5. Refrain from eating meat. Such foods contain lot of toxins secreted by animal during killing. Moreover, meat is considered Tamsik food with lot of negative energy.
6. Do occasional fasting with water and fruit juices. It will keep your system clean.
7. Relax and meditate regularly. Sitting postures of meditation (with straight spine) help a lot for balancing your pranic flow in the body.
8. Reduce time in watching TV, listening to Radio, reading newspapers and stray magazines. Excessive involvement in these things distract the mind and thereby affect the balance of energy body.
9. Go for regular walks in morning/evening in fresh air. Do moderate exercises and yogasanas with special emphasis on spinal exercises to keep it supple and straight.

10. Drink water stored in gold, silver or copper vessels. Water charged with these metals becomes filled with positive energy. Magnetized water is equally good.
11. Do pranayama or breathing exercises. They are very effective in balancing and strengthening your energy field. Specially develop the habit of rhythmic and diaphragmatic breathing as your moment to moment resting breathing. It has a very benevolent effect in maintaining a healthy aura.
12. Spend time with nature whenever you get opportunity. Take sunbath in the morning Fire element of our body is easily rejuvenated by sunbath.
13. Have regular water bath and do friction rubbing of body either by hand or by bath brush before bathing. Bathing in flowing river water is very good. Occasional bathing with salt water helps in cleasing the negative energy as salt has the characteristic of breaking down the negative energy. Among salts, sea salt is said to be especially useful.

    Some people do foot soaking in salt water. Water can be lukewarm, hot or cold depending upon your body's demand at a particular time. This is a very effective method for removing the negative energy of the body through the feet which is sucked by salt water. After foot soaking, this water should be thrown into W.C. because this water becomes impure after absorbing negativity.

    Foot soaking in salt water is said to clear our Swadhisthana and solar plexus chakra.
14. Walk barefoot on earth specially near river and countryside and on grass wet with morning dew. The earth element sucks lot of negativity through our feet and clear our Mooladhara chakra (or Root chakra). Sole chakra is an extension of Root chakra and is related directly to it. Sole chakra is also said to be related to Heart chakra.
15. Increase your awareness and attention in every task you do. This will increase your power and sensitivity to sense subtle impressions and sensations within and around you.

16. Laugh a lot. Loughing is a potent medicine for supplying you with instant positive energy. If you find difficult to laugh in your normal life routine, then read jokes in magazines/books, see comedy serials on TV, read entertainment columns of magazines etc. Also develop the habit of cutting and hearing jokes frequently (within limits of decency). Try to wear a natural smile on your face. This will keep you effortlessly positive.
17. Be aware of negative emotions (e.g. anger, fear, jealousy, hate, worry, impatience, hurry, revenge, etc.). Whenever they are arising in you, nip them in the bud at the very outset. Negative emotions throw your energy body completely out of balance.
18. Take some measures for keeping your home and work environment clean for creating a positives energy field as mentioned below:

(*i*) Evaporate pure camphor crystals. An easy way to do it is with the help of an electronic mosquito repellent. Place the camphor on a used mat. This way the camphor evaporates very slowly over many hours.

(*ii*) Burn incense ('Agarbatti's and Dhoops'). Their smell also purifies the energy of the surroundings.

(*iii*) Following oils have the power to create positive energy and neutralize negative energy. Hence burn oil lamp of the following oil:

(*a*) Mustard oil

(*b*) Sesame (Til) oil

(*c*) Ghee or clarified butter

(*iv*) Candle burning also neutralizes negative energy and creates positive energy. 'Trataka' on candle flame is very good because its light clears out the negative energy. This practice is said to clear Ajna Chakra.

(*v*) Salt water specially sea-salt water has great potential for neutralizing negative energy. One can mop the floor with sea-salt water or one can even keep a bowl of sea-salt water in a corner of the room. Every now and then put the bowl in the sun for a few hours and top it up and also change the water completely after certain days.

(*vi*) Fresh cut flowers with leaves and stems intact, placed in water in a vase or bowl and indoor plants are great positive energy generators and negative energy neutralizers. Yellow, orange and blue/violet flowers are quite good for this purpose.

(*vii*) Use those colours in your surroundings (room walls, curtains, carpet, furniture, wearing clothes) which promote positive energy and transmute negative energy. Such colours are white, blue, violet, green, yellow, orange, rose etc. Even visualizing these colours in meditation helps you in getting their positive energy.

(*viii*) Just like colours, there are certain sounds which generate positive energy and transmute negative energy. All satwik sounds and music come under this category. These sounds are found generally in old melodious songs and music, devotional songs, sould stirring bhajans, classical music, flute music, sound vibrations generated by blowing into a conch shell ('Shankh') and sounds simulating nature sounds e.g. sound of waterfall, flowing river, moving breeze, chirping of birds etc. By listening to such sounds, you always feel calm, centred, joyful and elevated. On the other hand, the modern Rajasik music like pop music only gives momentary thrill and excitement and hence it is not good for energy body.

(*ix*) Foodgrains, specially rice (uncooked), have the capacity to absorb and transmute negative energies. In particular, on the eleventh day of the waxing and waning moon cycle, this absorption is at a maximum. This day is called 'Ekadasi' (eleventh day). Hence they are kept in 'Pooja' (worship) places.

(*x*) Tulsi leaves are very effective in destroying the negative energy and purifying the atmosphere by creating positive energy. Hence always keep Tulsi plants in your terrace/ balcony.

(*xi*) Chanting of Mantras and Nam-Japas creates an energy pure environment mainly because of effect of pure sound vibrations. However, mental japa of mantras is equally effective in purifying the environment because the pure though vibrations created by mental japa also act on the energy atmosphere around because of the relationship between thought and life energy.

❑

42
BASIC RULES FOR GOOD HEALTH AND LONG LIFE

Combining an orderly, regulated way of life with observation of the five rules outlined below and regular shiatsu will help make life longer and more pleasant.

Proper Diet

Eating as much of everything your like is a diet that must be corrected. No matter how wholesome the foods you eat, balance must be maintained among them. First of all, it is essential to ensure enough of the three major energy foods proteins, fats, and carbohydrates–to facilitate an active life. In addition, the required amounts of minerals, water, and various vitamins needed to breakdown these foods and convert them into energy must be included in the diet.

Even with balanced menus, the body must be able to digest and assimilate the nutrients it takes in. Ensure that this is possible by eating at regular times in proper quantities and by chewing your food well. Breakfast is a must, even if it is only a small amount of highly nutritive food. Furthermore, the connection can cause upsets in the alimentary system. Avoid this by eating slowly and in a pleasant, calm atmosphere. This is all the more important since worry and irritation disrupt the functioning of the other internal organs as well.

Shiatsu on the abdomen improves the functioning of the stomach and intestines, thus stimulating digestion and absorption of nutrients. It may be self-administered.

Proper Sleep

Human beings sleep about one third of their lives if they take eight full hours of rest nightly. Sufficient sleep is more essential to recovery from fatigue than any therapy or drug. No matter how static one remains, as long as the body is awake, the organs continue to function; and the muscles preserve a state of tension. In sleep, however, the organs and the cerebral nerves rest; and the muscle relax, enabling the body to recover from weariness and be refreshed upon awakening.

There are many sleep patterns. The ideal one is falling asleep shortly after retiring, dropping into deep sleep soon thereafter and remaining in deep sleep until sleep gradually becomes increasingly shallow and waking occurs. This process can be compared to an aircraft that takes off immediately gains flight altitude, remains on altitude for the majority of the trip and gradually descends to land again at the destination point.

It is said that, though they are often forgotten, everyone has dreams every night. The level of sleep in which dreams occur is the rapid eye movement state, which is less desirable than deep sleep. Overindulgence in alcohol results in a sleeping state that is only half sleep and half intoxication. Since he does not enjoy restful, deep sleep, the person who has drunk too much often suffers from the state known as hangover on the morning after.

There is no doubt that "early to bed and early to rise" are linked with longevity. But the tempo of modern urban living makes it difficulat to follow the sound advice inherent in these words. Nonetheless, it is good to get up early in the morning and enjoy clean air before the pollution of daytime traffic has a chance to sully it. For a vigorous way of life, combine deep breathing of fresh morning air with a balanced diet, sound sleep, plenty of fresh air and regularly administered shiatsu.

Proper Elimination

Normally the bowels should move once a day, often immediately after breakfast. If this regimen is regularly observed, the alimentary system will function correctly; and nutrients will be readily absorbed.

The amount and nature of foods eaten determine the kinds and quantities of foeces eliminated. Excess consumption of difficult-to-digest foods causes either constipation or diarrhea. Psychological state too influence elimination.

To stay is good condition, eat a balanced diet regularly and perform self-administered abdominal shiatsu each morning. Upon waking, while lying on our back, press slowly on each of the points shown for from three to five seconds. Pressure should be applied with the palm of one hand. The other hand should be placed on top of the pressing hand. Repeat this as many times as seems necessary and then apply careful shiatsu pressure with three fingers to the area of the sigmoid colon to prevent constipation. Repeated daily, this therapy will restore appetite, improve digestion and regulate elimination. It will help prevent constipation in people who are inclined to this condition.

Proper Exercise

One of the most direct ways to prompt good health is proper energetic exercise combining leisure, work, and sports or some other active recreation. Human beings find a reason for living in purposeful, goal oriented activity; but in today's mechanized society, opportunities to display vitality are becoming increasing limited. Work is now subdivided and automated to the extent that human beings frequently do nothing but monotonous, repetitive operations. Means of transportation have become so convenient that people use their legs less than they should and prefer an elevator or escalator to even a moderate flight of steps. Under these conditions, it is scarcely surprising that people do not get enough exercise and that their muscular vigour declines. Recently, jogging has become popular with those who want to supplement their exercise or loose weight. But, without going this far, it is possible to achieve good results merely by walking more and moving the body as much as possible in ordinary daily activities. Walking is especially good, since it activates circulation in the legs and relieves sluggishness that inactivity causes. In addition, it is important to make full use of the bending, stretching, reaching and lifting that are parts of the movements performed in many apparently minor daily tasks.

From the shiatsu standpoint, I recommend special attention to exercising the hands and fingers. Small children who do not exercise these parts of the body enough fail to develop reflexes that could prevent injury in falls. Moving the hands and fingers develops the motor nerves that stimulate self protective reflex extensions of the hands and arms. I recommend encouraging children in the lower grades of primary school to administer shiatsu to themselves regularly. The shiatsu designed to strengthen the eyes and teeth is especially good since hand and finger exercises of this kind are related to cerebral functioning. The hand motions involved in painting, writing, playing the piano, or craft work have a good influence on powers of thought.

Laughter

Laughter is unique to the human being. A naturally laughing face is pleasing and beautiful. Physiologically, laughter is healthful and purifies the blood. In contrast anger and fear cause the face to become livid and creat pathological tensions in the internal organs. The up down-movement of the diaphragm caused by laughter stimulates the operation of the heart, improves the circulation and activates the functioning of the stomach and intestines. In addition, it helps regulate the internal secretions of the endocrine system.

A good laughter from the bottom of the belly once a day contributes to a better way of life. As the old sayings have it, "Laughter is the gate to happiness" and "A laugh rejuvenates, a frown ages."

❑

43
SYMBOLS OF REIKI

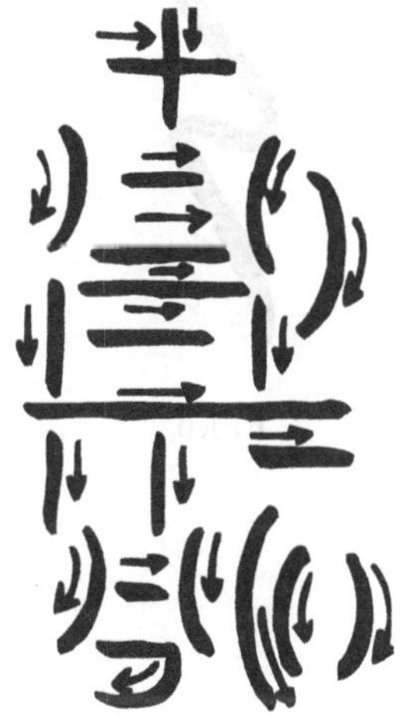

Hon Sha Ze Sho Nen

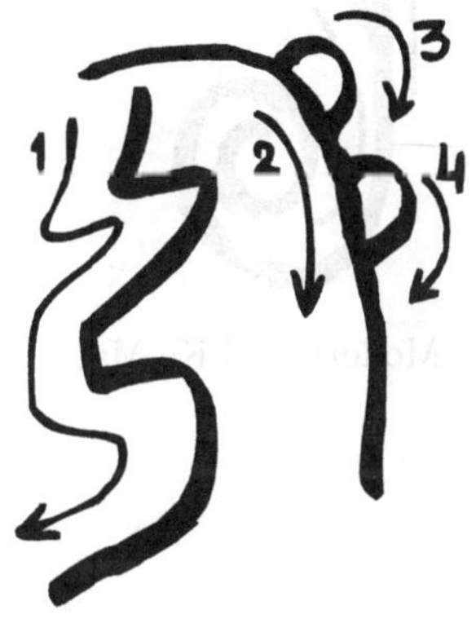

Sei He Ku

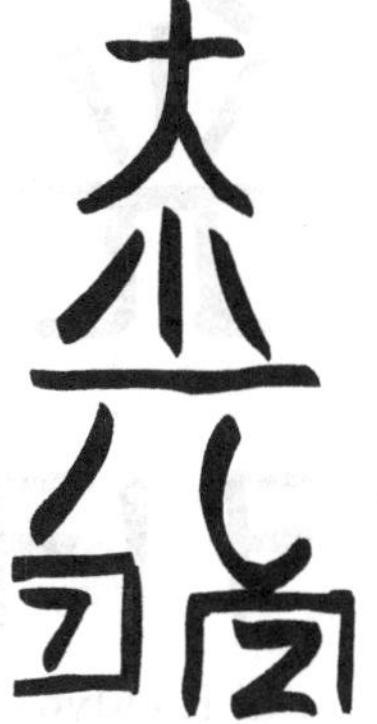

Dai Ko Myo (Variation)

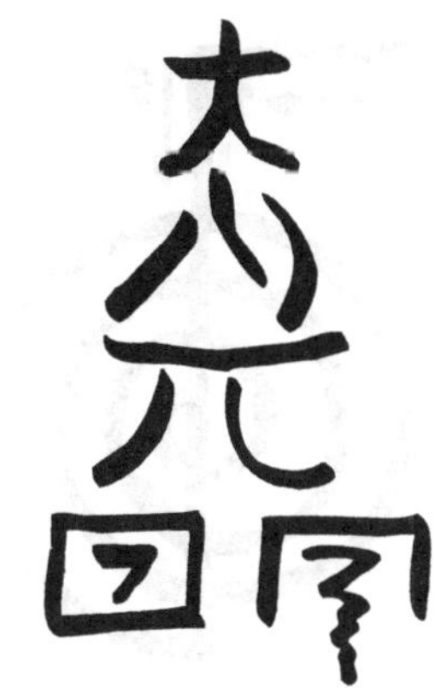

Dai Ko Myo
(Traditional Variation)

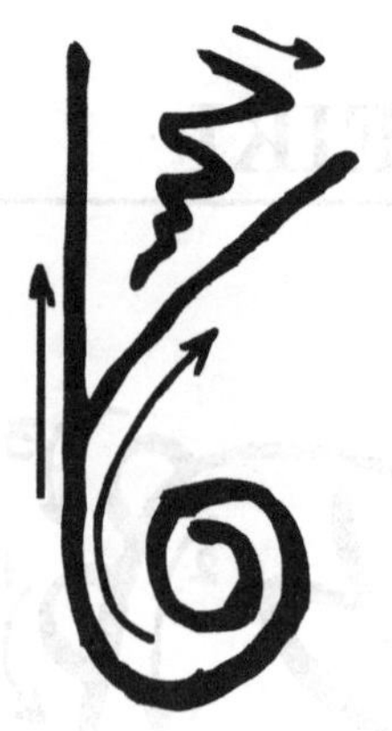

Modern Dai Ko Myo

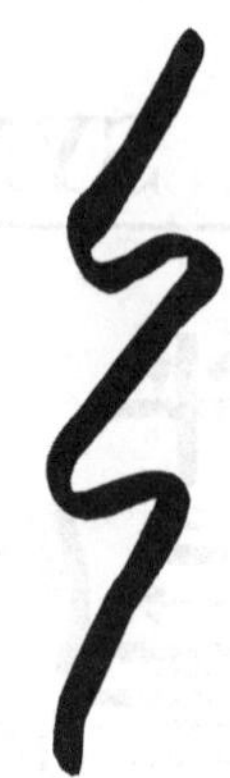

Raku

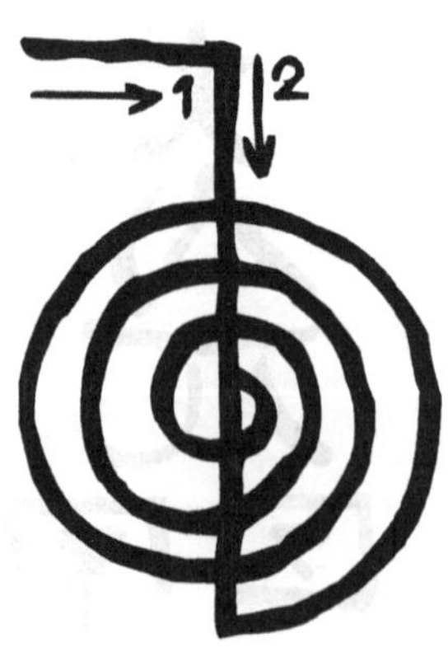

Cho Ku Rei

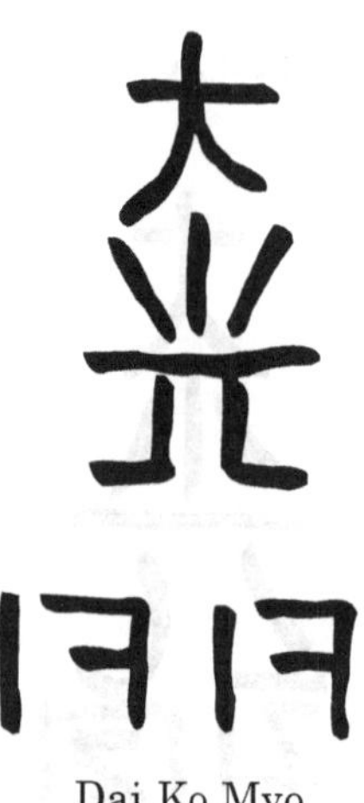

Dai Ko Myo

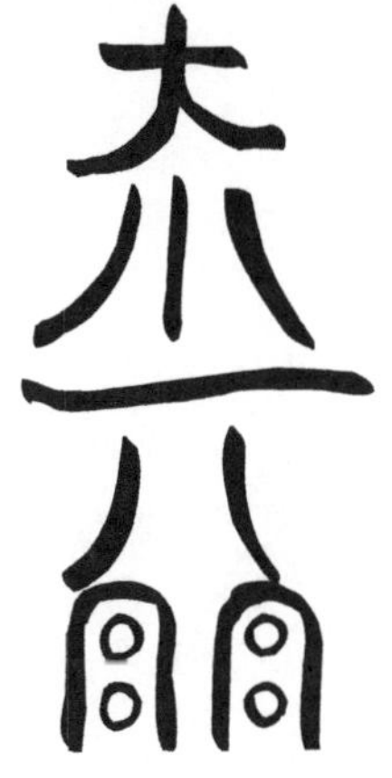

Dai Ko Myo (Variation)

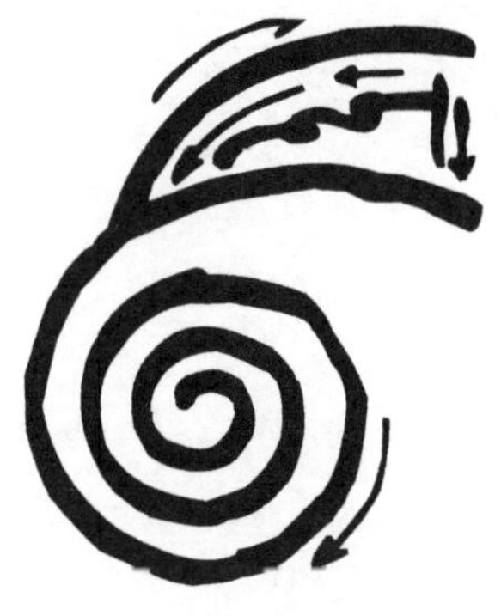

Modern Dai Ko Myo

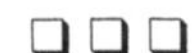

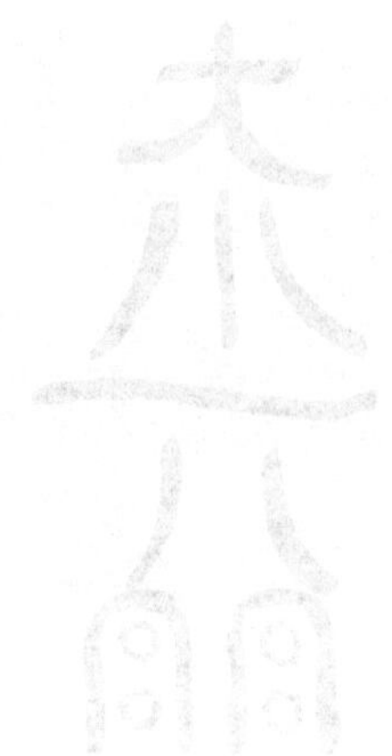